Cambridge Middle East Library

Medicine and power in Tunisia, 1780–1900

Cambridge Middle East Library

Medicine and power in Tunisia, 1780–1900

NANCY ELIZABETH GALLAGHER

DEPARTMENT OF HISTORY
UNIVERSITY OF CALIFORNIA, SANTA BARBARA

CAMBRIDGE UNIVERSITY PRESS

CAMBRIDGE
LONDON   NEW YORK   NEW ROCHELLE
MELBOURNE   SYDNEY

PUBLISHED BY THE PRESS SYNDICATE OF THE UNIVERSITY OF CAMBRIDGE
The Pitt Building, Trumpington Street, Cambridge, United Kingdom

CAMBRIDGE UNIVERSITY PRESS
The Edinburgh Building, Cambridge CB2 2RU, UK
40 West 20th Street, New York NY 10011–4211, USA
477 Williamstown Road, Port Melbourne, VIC 3207, Australia
Ruiz de Alarcón 13, 28014 Madrid, Spain
Dock House, The Waterfront, Cape Town 8001, South Africa

http://www.cambridge.org

First published 1983
First paperback edition 2002

A catalogue record for this book is available from the British Library

Library of Congress catalogue card number: 82-22163

ISBN 0 521 25124 9 hardback
ISBN 0 521 52939 5 paperback

Contents

Contents

Illustrations

In memory of Janet Lee Stevens,
scholar of the Egyptian and Tunisian theater
and friend of the Arab people.

Killed at the American Embassy in Beirut
on 18 April 1983 at the age of 32.

Acknowledgments

This study is the result of my interests in the social history of North Africa and in the interplay of cross-cultural medical ideas. I collected materials for the study in the archives, libraries, and bookshops of Tunis in 1974–5, began writing it at St Antony's College, Oxford, in 1976, and submitted the first version as a dissertation at the University of California, Los Angeles, in 1977. I completed the last lines of the second and final version while seated at the Funduq Husayn overlooking al-Azhar University, Cairo, in 1981. It was a pleasure to have begun the project in the *madina* (old city) of Tunis, where its historical events took place, and to have completed it at al-Azhar, where Islamic philosophies discussed in the text are still taught.

Experts in the field assisted at all stages of preparation. In Tunisia, Abdel-Jalil Temimi, editor, *Revue d'histoire maghrebine*, Mustafa Kraiem, Université de Tunis, Monceur Rouissi, Centre des recherches économiques et sociales, Paul Sebag, historian of Tunis, and Ahmad Ben Milad and Bou Bakr Ben Yahya, both medical historians of Tunis, generously made available archival materials and other unpublished sources, and shared with me their knowledge of history. Pères Fontaine and Magnin, Institut des belles lettres arabes, allowed me the use of their excellent library. Si Muhsin el Khoja, assistant at the archives for forty years, welcomed me warmly each day and courteously brought out dossier after dossier.

At Oxford, Albert Hourani guided the early stages of the study with great insight and expertise. I shall never forget his kindness nor the dignified and historic atmosphere of Oxford. Norman Cigar read and commented upon the manuscript with an eye for precision and detail.

At U.C.L.A., Afaf Lutfi al-Sayyid Marsot was an exemplary teacher and dissertation director. Robert Frank, Judith and Peter Gran, and Dunning Wilson constructively criticized the first version. Andrea Ball improved the dissertation with thoughtful editing. During the final revisions, the following scholars offered major and minor suggestions: Abdel Rahman Ayoub, Jacques Berque, Nikki Keddie, Speros Vryonis, and Stanley Yoder. Ralph Jaeckel helped bring into focus the central lines of the study. Teresa Ruggieri Joseph recommended substantial structural changes in the text. Colleen Trujillo skillfully prepared the final copy while I was 10,000 miles away in Egypt.

In France, Lucette Valensi and François Arnoulet discussed the project with me. Michael Dols, California State University, Hayward, LaVerne Kuhnke, Northeastern University, Boston, and Joel Montague, Population Council, told me of their research on related topics. Jere Bacharach, University of Washington, Kenneth L. Brown, University of Manchester, Leon Carl Brown, Princeton University, Carlo Cipolla, University of California, Berkeley, and Timothy Mitchell, Princeton University, read all or part of the final manuscript and offered advice resulting in revisions and clarifications.

My parents followed the project with great interest and traveled to both Tunis and Cairo while I was there. Tony Gardner was helpful and supportive at all times.

Earlier stages were funded by a Fulbright–Hayes Dissertation Fellowship and by a two-year fellowship from the Josiah Macy Foundation for the History of Medicine and Biological Sciences. Final revisions were made possible with funding and sabbatical leave provided by the Academic Senate and by the Department of History, University of California, Santa Barbara. Diana Lorenz, Department of Geography, U.C. Santa Barbara, drew the maps. I am grateful to these and other persons for their assistance. I of course take full responsibility for the historical accuracy and analyses.

N.E.G.

Note on transliteration

Transliteration of Arabic words and names follows the system of the *International Journal of Middle East Studies*. Macrons and diacritic marks are dropped in the text but included in the Glossary, where most Arabic terms in the text are defined and fully transliterated. I have in general used the familiar spellings of place names, most of which have come into English via French. For lesser-known places I have used simplified Arabic transliteration.

Abbreviations

A.G.G.T.
Archives Générales du Gouvernement Tunisien, Dar al-Bey, Ministry of Foreign Affairs, Tunis.

Annales, E.S.C.
Annales, economie, société, civilisation.

Bin Diyaf
Ahmad Ibn Abi Diyaf, *Ithaf ahl al-zaman bi akhbar muluk tunis wa 'ahd al-aman*, 8 vols. (Tunis, 1963–6).

Desfontaines
J.A. Peyssonnel and R.L. Desfontaines, *Voyages dans les régences de Tunis et d'Alger*, Vol. II (Paris, 1838).

Ferrini, *Intorno al cholera*
G. Ferrini, *Intorno al cholera di Tunisi dell'anno 1867* (Milan, 1868).

F.O.
Public Record Office, correspondence between British consuls in Tunis and Foreign Office, London.

Frank, 'Tunis'
L. Frank, 'Tunis', in *L'Univers, histoire et description de tous les peuples : Algérie, Etats Tripolitains, Tunis* (Paris, 1850), pp. 3–143.

Ganiage, *Origines*
J. Ganiage, *Les Origines du protectorat français en Tunisie, 1863–1881* (Paris, 1959).

Kitab al-bashi
Hamuda Ibn 'Abd al-'Aziz, *Kitab al-bashi*, Pt I (Tunis, 1970); complete MSS Nos. 1236 and 1249 (British Museum).

Lumbroso, *Cenni sul cholera*
A. Lumbroso, *Cenni storico-scientifici sul cholera-morbus asiatico che invase la reggenza di Tunis nel 1849–1850* (Marseilles, 1850).

Masson
P. Masson, *Histoire des établissements et du commerce français dans l'Afrique barbaresque, 1560–1793* (Paris, 1903).

Mechra et Melki	M. Seghir ben Youssef, *Mechra et Melki: chronique tunisienne, 1705–1771* (Tunis, 1900).
Peyssonnel	J.A. Peyssonnel and R.L. Desfontaines, *Voyages dans les régences de Tunis et d'Alger*, Vol. I (Paris, 1838).
Plantet, *Correspondance*	E. Plantet, *Correspondance des beys de Tunis et des consuls de France avec la cour, 1577–1830*, 3 vols. (Paris, 1893–9).
Safwat al-i'tibar	M. Bayram al-Khamis, *Safwat al-i'tibar bi mustawda al-amsar wa al-aqtar*, Vol. II, Bk 2 (Beirut, 1972–3).
Valensi, *Fellahs tunisiens*	L. Valensi, *Fellahs tunisiens: l'économie rurale et la vie des campagnes aux XVIIIᵉ et XIXᵉ siècles* (Paris, 1977).

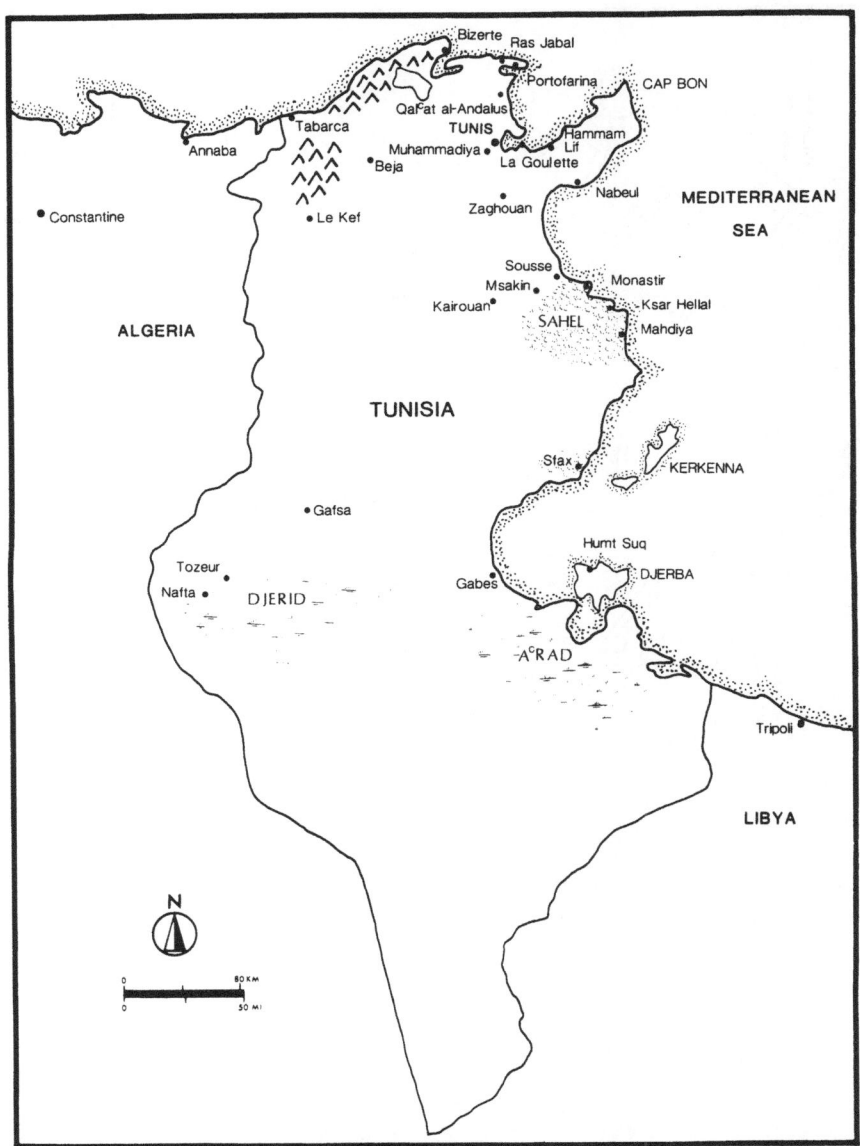

Map 1. Tunisia

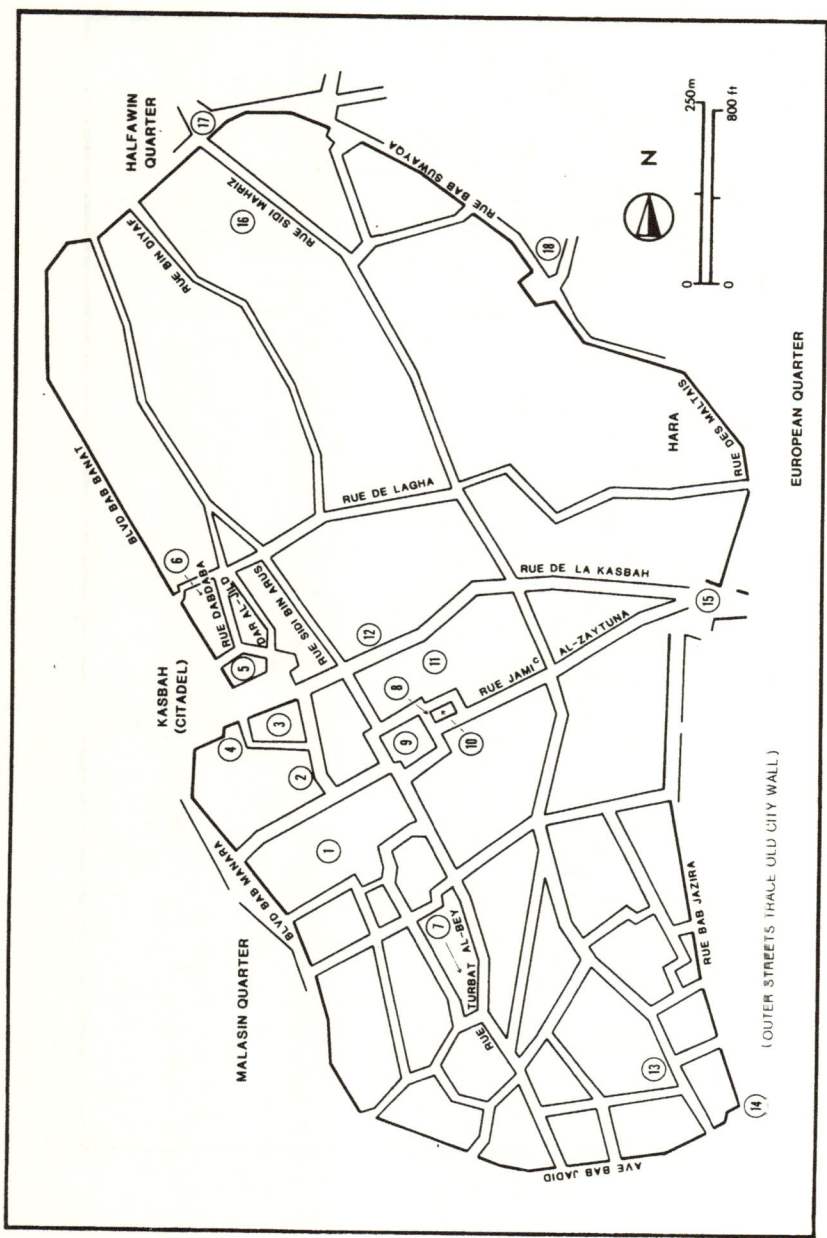

Map 2. The contemporary medina of Tunis

① CARPET SUQ (MARKET) ② JEWELRY SUQ ③ DAR AL-BEY ARCHIVES ④ SADIQI HOSPITAL ⑤ GOVERNMENT BUILDINGS ⑥ TAKIYA ⑦ TURBAT AL-BEY ⑧ MEDICINAL HERB SHOPS ⑨ GREAT MOSQUE (JAMI' AL-ZAYTUNA) ⑩ NATIONAL LIBRARY ('ATTARINE) ⑪ PERFUME SUQ ⑫ MARISTAN ⑬ SUQ OF TANNERS ⑭ BAB JAZIRA ⑮ BAB AL-BAHR ⑯ MOSQUE OF SIDI MAHRIZ ⑰ BAB SUWAYQA ⑱ BAB CARTHAGE

Introduction

Method and approach

At the beginning of the nineteenth century, Louis Frank, a French doctor practicing in Tunis, found that he had to stay on good terms with the Muslim chief of physicians to practice European medicine without difficulties. At the end of the century, Hamda b. Kilani, a Muslim doctor and son of the former chief of physicians of Tunis, found that he had to be classed as *médecin toléré* (a second-class medical status) by the French medical authority to practice Arabic medicine at all. Why the change in power?

The answer emerges in the long struggle between Arabic and European medicine that accelerated with European economic expansion. The intricacies of the medical confrontation are best seen through the history of the major epidemics that struck the people of Tunisia between 1780 and 1900. The epidemics threatened the lives of vast numbers of people and called forth responses from all levels of society: ordinary people, medical personnel, religious authorities, and the political and commercial elite. The process of medical change revealed by the epidemics can only be studied meaningfully against the political, social, and economic realities of the times.

In Tunisia, the shift from Arabic to European medicine was a fundamental part of the colonial experience. The suspicion of the Muslim elite that European science contained superior sources of knowledge and therefore of temporal power led them to reconsider long-held medical concepts and to undertake a reform program with both enthusiasm and misgiving. The indigenous government adopted new policies regarding disease and its prevention during the intense struggle between Muslim and European civilization. Toward the end of the nineteenth century, French colonialists in Tunisia came to see medicine as a fundamental tool of their 'civilizing mission' which could, through its humanitarian results, serve the political interests of France.

While medical subjects rarely appear in standard sources – Arabic chronicles, consular letters, and archival materials – records of epidemics were often considered important enough to be written down and saved. Quarantine notices, commercial registers, and military reports from provincial authorities all contained occasional references to outbreaks of epidemics. In addition, most travelers mentioned epidemics that occurred during their travels, and European doctors practicing in Tunisia wrote books and articles about their experiences with them. From these primary sources emerges a story of social struggle not only with disease but with the new challenges presented by European expansion.

Earlier medical historians occasionally traced the course of an epidemic, justifying their projects by the intrinsic interest in one aspect of local history or, in a wider sense, of the human experience. In recent years, however, social historians have begun studying epidemics, using new theoretical approaches which combine ecological, epidemiological, medical, and demographic information with more conventional historical source materials. Most studies of epidemics contain several analytical approaches to the material, but three major historical approaches can be distinguished.

The first views disease and especially epidemic diseases as causative agents in history, resulting in the fall of empires and the decline of civilizations. William McNeill, in his *Plagues and Peoples* (1976), theorizes that smallpox facilitated the Spanish conquest of the Americas because the Amerindians, seeing the Spanish survive while they themselves were decimated by the mysterious disease, may have concluded that the enemy possessed special magical powers. The author expands his observations, speculating on the varied effects of infectious diseases on the course of human affairs worldwide and over long periods of time. Michael Dols, in *The Black Death in the Middle East* (1977), advances the thesis that the plague of 1347 and its resulting population decline led directly to the crises of the Mamluk Sultanate in the later fourteenth and fifteenth centuries. Historians of medieval Europe have extensively debated this issue: the many facets of the argument are summarized in W. Bowsky, ed., *The Black Death: A Turning Point in History?* (1971). The debate on plague and its historic consequences is one aspect of a larger dialogue on whether or not demographic forces are the fundamental ones in historical change.

The second approach sees epidemics as mirrors or magnifying glasses reflecting and revealing underlying social forces and conflicts and changes in values and attitudes that might normally escape the historian's eye. Louis Chevalier, for example, in *Classes laborieuses et classes dangereuses à Paris pendant la première moitié du XIXe siècle* (1958), portrays social tensions and resentments in France through the cholera riots that occurred in the poorer quarters of Paris, where the disease struck most severely. Charles Rosenberg, in *The Cholera Years* (1962), traces the 'dissipation of piety' and the development of a 'positivistic temper of thought and expression' in the United States through the cholera epidemics that struck in 1832, 1849, and 1866. Carlo Cipolla, in *Cristofano and the Plague* (1973) and *Faith, Reason, and the Plague in Seventeenth-Century Tuscany* (1979), depicts the emotions, attitudes, and behavior of various segments of society in seventeenth-century Italy through the communal responses to plague.

The third approach demonstrates changes in medical theories and practices as seen through and resulting from societal experience with epidemics. Severe diseases call for some sort of medical action; how and why do medical ideas change over time? Roderick McGrew's *Russia and the Cholera* (1965) describes the development of liberal, sophisticated medical writings that paralleled developments in contemporary Russian literature through the events of the cholera epidemic of 1823–32. Margaret Pelling, in *Cholera, Fever, and English Medicine, 1825–1865* (1978), traces the intellectual development of epidemiological theories in England that led to public concern about medical dilemmas previously thought private.

These three approaches to epidemics and history are all included in the following study. The first approach, regarding the role of mortality as the determinant of historical advance or decline, is critically evaluated following discussion of the epidemics. The second approach, illustrating the internal dynamics of a given society through popular response to epidemic disease, reveals Muslim and European communal relationships that shifted as the balance of economic and political power changed. The third approach, discussing medical development through a society's experiences with epidemics, shows how the epidemics hastened the transition from Arabic to European medical institutions. Moreover, European-style medical reform, completed in Tunis at governmental levels by 1900, was used as a major justification of the colonial system that operated in North Africa.

Plague, cholera, and typhus

In the Muslim world and in the West severe epidemic diseases periodically swept across the land terrorizing and decimating the inhabitants. Each civilization tried desperately to protect itself against such diseases but until the late nineteenth century, Muslim and European medical efforts alike generally proved futile. Medical ideas about epidemics in both regions originated from religious concepts of causation, empirical observations, and Greek and Islamic scholarly traditions. Ideas concerning prevention and treatment were often contradictory but remained relatively constant from antiquity until the nineteenth century, when positivist scientific inquiry and new political and social interests largely negated them. The three epidemic diseases that struck Tunisia most severely during the period under study, 1780–1900, were plague, cholera, and typhus. All three caused fundamental rethinking of received tradition on the part of the Muslim elite in the context of European scientific, commercial, and political impact.

By 1800 plague to most Europeans was a distant memory associated with medieval times. The last major epidemic in England had occurred in 1664–5 and was immortalized by Daniel Defoe in *A Journal of the Plague Year* (1722). Marseilles was stricken by severe plague epidemics in 1705 and 1720 but after that time the disease seemed to disappear from France. It lingered on, however, in North Africa and the Middle East until the early nineteenth century and in the Far East until the early twentieth century. With its horrifying symptoms, high fatality rates, and massive epidemic nature, plague gripped the popular imagination. Arabic and Latin medical manuscripts had lengthy sections on plague, whereas other diseases were often less extensively discussed. Plague struck the Middle East and Europe with equal severity, and each region had long-standing philosophical controversies and medical theories concerning the proper method of defense.

Bubonic plague, the most common form of the disease, is characterized by swelling of the lymph nodes (buboes, in the armpits and groin), blackening of the skin, fever, chills, nausea, and delirium. Its cause was unknown until 1894, when the bacillus, *Yersinia pestis*, was discovered nearly simultaneously by two researchers working independently in Hong Kong, Alexander Yersin and Shibasaboro Kitasato. Although people often noticed rats dying in large numbers prior to an outbreak of plague, no one suspected the connection. Now it is known that fleas, especially rat fleas, are generally responsible for the transmission of bubonic plague. From time to time rodent fleas become infected and transmit the disease to their hosts, such as rats or squirrels. The hosts die and the fleas seek other hosts, including human beings.

Two other forms of plague are also caused by *Yersinia pestis*. Pneumonic plague is contracted when the bacillus is transmitted directly from person to person by means of the respiratory channel. Septicemic plague results when the bacillus is introduced directly into the bloodstream by fleabite. In both forms the characteristic buboes are absent, confusing diagnosis, and fatality rates are higher than for bubonic plague. Pneumonic and septicemic forms sometimes appeared during severe bubonic plague epidemics. In the 1930s and 1940s it was learned that plague is susceptible to antibiotics such as streptomycin and tetracycline.

Why plague has disappeared in epidemic form in modern times is a matter of controversy. Among the explanations are improved quarantine procedures that prevent contact with infected persons, cotton, or grain; improved building procedures that reduce the proximity of rats to man; a shift from the black house rat to the less domesticated brown rat; public rather than private storage of grain, which reduces contact with rat fleas that breed in wheat chaff; an increase in human immunity to *Yersinia pestis*; increased human resistance through improved nutrition; and medical advances that effectively isolate and treat the infected. Each explanation can be partially disproved by detailed local studies, though perhaps their cumulative effects have been decisive to date. A complete and satisfactory explanation of the recent absence of plague epidemic has yet to be made.[1]

Two major plague epidemics struck Tunisia during the period covered by this study, in 1784 and 1818. Each lasted for many months, devastating the populace, but no plague has occurred since. Chapter 1 deals with these two epidemics and their social and economic consequences in the historical context of the time.

Cholera, the second disease considered in this study, was the most dreaded disease of the nineteenth century. Cholera had apparently existed endemically in India for centuries. In 1817 it began to spread to other regions in epidemic form, perhaps aided by improved means of transportation developed during the Industrial Revolution. In 1817 cholera reached the Arabian peninsula, Iran, Turkey, southern Russia, Thailand, and Japan. Everywhere it killed thousands, with whole families succumbing within hours or days. By the mid-1820s the disease had spread through central Europe and appeared in England in 1831 and in the United States in 1832. Some six pandemics, or world epidemics, struck during the nineteenth century. Mecca and Medina, centers of pilgrimage from India, southeast Asia, the Middle East, and Africa, were important centers of cholera transmission.[2]

Like plague, cholera is a fearful disease. It strikes its victims suddenly: within hours a healthy person falls ill and experiences uncontrollable vomiting and diarrhea. In extreme cases, the skin color turns from blue to black as the victim dehydrates and appears to age before one's eyes. Fatality rates in the nineteenth century were between 40 and 60 percent in most regions. No known medical treatment was successful against the new disease. Traditional treatments such as bleeding and new remedies such as electric shock were tried in vain. In Tunis, as in many European cities, people sometimes suspected doctors of spreading the disease to kill

5

off poor people, or of being in the pay of the government, which hoped to divert attention from opposition to it by creating public alarm. Hospitals and doctors' care were widely feared as sure sentences as death. Cholera killed by dehydrating its victims, and the bleedings and purges prescribed by doctors were thought to hasten death.[3]

Cholera caused a crisis of confidence in the nineteenth-century European medical profession, then in the midst of the Scientific Revolution, and precipitated an avalanche of publications reporting investigation of the disease. New medical efforts to treat cholera, however, failed. Despite the unknown cause, the connection between poor sanitation and the incidence of cholera soon became apparent. In London in 1854 the contagiousness of the disease, much in dispute at the time, was convincingly established during a localized outbreak. John Snow, a medical doctor and researcher, went to the scene of the outbreak and learned that all of the victims had drunk from the same well. He removed the pump handle and the epidemic stopped. The cause of the disease was not determined for another thirty years, when Robert Koch isolated the causative bacillus, *Vibrio cholerae*, in Egypt. Snow's discovery and similar observations elsewhere stimulated public health reforms in European and Middle Eastern cities.[4]

Today, cholera patients usually recover with rehydration often aided by antibiotics and general hospital care. Epidemics still strike the Mediterranean and other regions of the world, however, occasionally impeding travel, and if immediate medical care is not obtainable, causing deaths.

Cholera has invaded Tunisia many times; the most severe epidemics during the period under study came in 1849 and in 1867. Cholera was a new disease to Muslims and Europeans, and each group hoped to learn the means of prevention and treatment from the other. Chapters 2 and 3 discuss the events of these major epidemics and the dialogue among political and medical authorities who tried to deal with the crises on their own, often conflicting, terms.

Typhus, the third disease considered in this study, first spread in Europe in epidemic form during the wars of the fifteenth century. It is commonly found among those unable to avail themselves of normal hygiene – prisoners, refugees, and military troops. The disease was particularly virulent during the Thirty Years War of 1618–48. Typhus was responsible for the deaths of most of the 600,000 troops lost during Napoleon's famous retreat from Moscow in 1812–13.

Symptoms of the disease include a spotted rash, nausea, chills, and fever. The fatality rate ranges from about 5 percent among children to 25 percent among young adults, and 50 percent among the aged. Charles

Nicolle discovered the mode of transmission while working in the Sadiqi hospital of Tunis in 1909. He noticed that patients recently admitted to the hospital spread the disease to others but that once patients were bathed and their clothing changed, no more cases occurred. He surmised that the body louse was the vector, and additional experimentation confirmed his observation. The causative agent, a virus, was discovered by Stanislaus von Prowazek in 1914 and by Henrique da Rocha-Lima in 1916. The virus was named *Rickettsia prowazekii* after von Prowazek and Howard T. Ricketts, who died investigating the disease. In 1939 the insecticide properties of DDT were discovered and the chemical was widely used as a delousing powder by Allied troups during World War II. Today typhus patients usually recover with symptomatic treatment, proper nutrition, and hospital care.[5]

Typhus appeared frequently in Tunisia; owing to its association with the famine and cholera which preceded it, the epidemic of 1868 was exceptionally destructive. This epidemic, which is studied in Chapter 3, followed the famine and cholera of 1866 and 1867 and directly preceded bankruptcy and the beginning of direct European economic domination.

Arabic and European concepts of epidemic disease, c. 1800

Prior to the twentieth century, effective treatment of these diseases remained a mystery. Since earliest times, however, people tried to find ways to deal with such threats to life. Muslims and Europeans alike tried preventive and curative measures based on empirical observations, ancient medical theories, and religious traditions. Evil spirits were widely suspect as the cause of epidemics. Genies that pricked victims with plague-poisoned arrows figured in the Old and New Testaments and in the Quran. Until the end of the eighteenth century, the wearing of amulets during time of plague was common throughout the Middle East and Europe. Muslims and Christians sometimes considered plague a punishment for sin requiring prayers and invocations for deliverance.

During the Black Death of 1348, it was clear that plague spread from region to region and port to port. Trading cities of the Italian peninsula, in frequent contact with other regions, began to institute quarantines on ships and land and sea travelers, isolating the sick and disinfecting cargoes. By the seventeenth century, many European cities had adopted some form of quarantining when plague was announced elsewhere.[6] In the Ottoman Empire the practice was less prevalent, but Istanbul and Tunis had quarantined ships since at least the early eighteenth century.

Arabic medical theories in 1800 were derived from two major sources of medical authority: Galenic (Greek)–Islamic medicine and prophetic medicine. Galenic–Islamic medicine, exemplified in the writings of Ibn Sina (d. 1037), held that disease was caused by an imbalance of the four humors of the body: hot, cold, moist, and dry. The primary elements in the balance were blood, mucous, yellow bile, and black bile, respectively, matters of the four humors. An individual had a characteristic humoral balance manifested as a sanguine, phlegmatic, choleric, or melancholic temperament according to the predominant humor. When illness struck, the balance was upset and the doctor's role was to correct it. In early-nineteenth-century Tunis, for example, a Muslim doctor once diagnosed a fever which he thought was caused by 'accretion of blood in the pituitary'.[7] The remedy was to remove the excess blood by bleeding the patient. Excess phlegm could cause 'cold' illnesses like influenzas, for which hot foods were prescribed.

In eighteenth-century North Africa hot foods such as ginger, pennyroyal, garlic, nutmeg, cloves, honey, and nuts were thought to quicken the blood and to loosen the joints. Cold foods such as vinegar, cucumbers, oranges, watermelons, and turnips made the skin cool and the body still. For a general fortifier, hot foods such as honey, milk, and ground sesame were boiled, filtered, and taken each morning. For 'epidemic fever' one took cooling herbs or roots. For extended fevers, one ate bread made of barley and wheat and drank a potion of ground bark and pomegranate leaves mixed with sugar extracted from ground ginger, hummus (chickpeas) boiled with mastic, and lupin. The patient's room was filled with vapors of burning willow leaves to disinfect the air.[8]

Prophetic medicine, the second major influence in eighteenth-century Muslim medical theory and practice, was based on medical customs prevailing in Muhammad's time in the towns and deserts of the Arabian peninsula. Such practices were sanctified in numerous sayings and traditions (*hadith*s) about the words and deeds of Muhammad and his family and companions. In one famous hadith the Prophet acknowledged three cures: honey, scarification, and cautery.[9] In other hadiths, a black grain (possibly cumin), Indian aloes, and camel's milk and urine are mentioned as remedies and were widely used by Muslim healers. Scarification and cautery became basic surgical treatments throughout the Islamic world.[10]

Scarification was performed by first applying surface pressure to cause the skin to swell; then a small knife with a long curved blade heated red hot at the tip was lightly touched repeatedly to the sick area in lines or configurations. When the scarification was completed, the doctor rolled a baton over the scratches to stop the bleeding. To treat stomach ailments, the stomach region was lightly scarified or scratched; for a sprained limb the appropriate muscle was scarified.[11] To this day many

Tunisians, in the case of an injury, lightly scratch the affected area with a razor, releasing a bit of blood, and claim to feel much better afterward.

Cautery was a means of treating superficial wounds and skin ailments. Rings of hot iron, for example, were lightly placed around bullet wounds. Sometimes infected sores such as plague buboes were cauterized with branding irons. Many famous hadiths and proverbs reinforced these remedies: 'fire draws out the poison of the nerves'; 'the best medicine is cautery'. Infections were thought to be caused by bodily impurities that could be treated mechanically.[12]

Phlebotomy, or bleeding, was an important component of Galenic–Islamic and prophetic medicine. In medieval times, it was developed into a complex art of surgery of the veins widely practiced in North Africa. Bleeding was most commonly done from small blood vessels in the nostril or earlobe but also at the location of injury or pain. Many cultures have suspected excess blood to be a cause or symptom of disease.[13]

Whereas Galenic–Islamic medicine generally attributed disease solely to natural causes, prophetic medicine ascribed disease to divine power and the actions of evil spirits (usually referred to as *jinn*) as well as to natural causes such as cold wind. Jinn were considered susceptible to a variety of substances, amulets, and the interference of persons possessing *baraka* (mystic power). Baraka was thought to be inherited by certain descendants of the Prophet, or possessed by marabouts (Arabic, *murabitun* [in North Africa, holy men or women, saints]). Jinn were believed capable of covering great distances in an instant and, though usually invisible, they were able to assume human or animal form, to live in marshy places, and to frequent people's homes. Gases and bad odors were manifestations of jinn; when walking near foul miasmas or latrines one asked protection from them. They were thought to be especially active during the cool evening hours. Unpredictable, they became vengeful or violent if offended by those who shared their world. Retaliation often came in the form of an illness; if one stepped on a jinn and failed to mitigate the offense by one of the available means, the result might be a mild illness or an injury. For more serious offenses, jinn might take over the whole body and produce symptoms of mental illness, epilepsy, madness, or depression. Armies of jinn attacking in swarms could cause epidemic disease.[14]

Substances believed to cancel the evil effects of jinn included sunlight, salt, silver, gunpowder, henna, kohl, and the fumes of strong substances such as tar and pungent herbs. Since it was believed that epidemic diseases were caused by armies of jinn, one logical means of individual protection was an amulet (*hajib*) prepared by a marabout and 'purchased' for a donation of a few cents or a small gift. Amulets came in many forms.

Among the more common were papers that contained sacred words or numbers. When attaching the amulet to his or her clothing, the patient was to recite a formula such as 'God the all-powerful, the creator, the master of bodies and souls, cure me.' Sometimes the papers were placed in a cup of water to dissolve the ink and the potion was drunk.[15]

Prophetic medical procedures for dealing with the spirits were further developed by men and women of the Sufi orders. Exorcizing the jinn was a formal ritual with prescribed methods which varied from order to order. Sufi hospices functioned like hospitals in the sense that those seeking cure might stay in them until the healing power of the marabout took effect. Still performed in North Africa, the ceremonies resemble modern group therapy sessions in that the sufferer is supported by a community of well-wishers who direct their efforts toward his or her recovery. If cured, a patient might acquire a new identity as a follower of the saint and a member of the Sufi order.[16]

One of the largest Sufi orders in Tunisia was the 'Isawa order, which specialized in healing ceremonies. The order was founded in about 1500 in southern Morocco and spread eastward. The founder of the order, Muhammad b. 'Isa, was famous for his cures – laying on of hands and spraying saliva – and was thought to be immune to disease and to have passed this immunity to his followers, who were called in to perform the healing ceremonies in time of epidemic. The 'Isawa were thought to draw the jinn away from the susceptible lay persons to themselves. To heal a sick person, the 'Isawa recited specific formulas, massaged or placed snakes (friendly creatures) near the patient, or, like the founder, passed their hands over the sick person while reciting the name of God, the Prophet, and 'Isa. In ceremonies designed to cure a patient possessed by jinn, the 'Isawa joined hands in a circle and danced to flute and drum music, jerking forward and backward and repeating the *shahada* (profession of faith). When worked into a frenzy, they devoured scorpions and broken glass, walked on coals, swallowed swords, and attacked things colored black or persons wearing black, horror of black being a characteristic of the order.[17]

Similar healing practices exist in many parts of the world. The 'mediators with spirits', when in a state of possession, salivate, roll their eyes, become indifferent to pain, and can perform feats impossible in a normal state. Generally, rhythmic chanting, motion, music, and sometimes hallucinogenic drugs help to produce this state. The cures have been witnessed many times; modern advocates of the art of exorcism attribute their effectiveness to magnetic forces of unknown nature, and above all the confidence, will, and conviction of the patient.[18]

In Tunisia, the elite tended to consider such practices excessive, magical, and un-Islamic. Individuals of all classes, however, sought cures from secular and religious healers trained in the art of medicine. For serious diseases or injuries, selection of medical system was often a question of ability to pay, with an occasional but not universal preference for European medicine.

European medical theories in 1800 were also derived from Galenic–Islamic sources, but during the Enlightenment and the Scientific Revolution, as a result of new methods of experimental research, new chemicals had been added to European pharmacology, anatomical knowledge had been advanced, and certain diseases had been differentiated and classified. Medical instruments were more numerous and more complex and there was great enthusiasm for medical and biological research. Effective means of prevention and treatment of most diseases, however, were to remain uncertain for many years. In 1800 Europeans suspected three general causes of epidemic disease: miasma, contagion, and astral influence (all of which orginated in antiquity). Miasmas were corruptions of the air, usually believed to be caused by putrefying matter or decomposing bodies. Contagion was thought to be a kind of material from an infected person that could cause disease. It was vaguely referred to as 'fomites', coated with a substance rather like glue that could attach to the victim. Astral influences referred to planetary actions that were thought to influence the course of events and accordingly the spread of disease. Many believed in all three causes or in a combination of them and thought divine power ultimately responsible for their actual operation. But by the beginning of the nineteenth century theories of astrological or divine causation were nearly dropped by the medical profession. In time of epidemic, however, ordinary people demonstrated their belief in contagion by terrorized flight from the diseased.

Following the Marseilles plague epidemic of 1720–1, doctors debated whether plague and certain other infectious diseases were in fact contagious. M. Chirac, personal physician of the Regent of France, went to Marseilles with a commission to investigate the nature of the disease. The commission disagreed but the majority opted for the contagionist line. Chirac, head of the commission, himself was an anticontagionist; in his published writings he accounted for the immunity of a girls' convent located in the center of Marseilles during the 1720 plague by their faith in God. In 1724, as will be shown in Chapter 1, he sent Peyssonnel, one of the Marseilles doctors, to Tunis to learn whether the Muslims thought plague contagious and how they treated it.

In 1721, on the basis of information about the Marseilles epidemic, an English physician, Richard Mead, published his influential *Short Discourse Concerning Pestilential Contagion* in which he argued that plague was imported in goods such as cotton, by diseased persons, or by air. The air could be modified by atmospheric changes, a concept derived from miasmic theories. To Mead, plague was a poison that originated in Asia or Africa and quarantines then in use should be reinforced.[19]

Yet it was observed that individuals, families, or whole quarters were inexplicably spared the effects of a given epidemic, and even the most strictly enforced quarantine rarely succeeded in containing disease spread. Doctors who treated plague victims often did not contract the disease. Furthermore, plague occurred seasonally, disappearing in winter. A succession of anticontagionists argued that plague was an exhalation (miasma) that originated in the ground, was extracted by the heat of the sun, and was carried by winds. Though miasmas were thought to come from Asia or Africa, quarantines against them were quite useless.

The controversy between miasmists and contagionists was of critical significance because quarantines disrupted orderly trade and commerce, causing economic losses that seemed at times more severe than the disease itself. In the early nineteenth century the debates between contagionists and miasmists were to become more heated. Clot Bey, Muhammad 'Ali's director of health in Egypt and a leading anti-contagionist, speculated that plague was caused by 'electro-magnetic disturbances operating quite independently of local insanitation or infection'.[20] Some thought plague and typhus were different symptomatic manifestations of one communicable disease that could transform itself according to changes in climate or other natural conditions. The debates on miasmic or contagionist causation excluded such clearly contagious diseases as smallpox and focused on other major scourges of the nineteenth century: plague, typhoid, typhus, yellow fever, and cholera. In 1700 few doctors had totally abandoned the humoral theory of disease. But by 1800 the practice of systematic recording of observations, drawing of inferences from recorded data, and testing of inferences with controls led researchers to question ancient medical concepts of causation. However, lacking the germ theory of disease, treatments developed in antiquity remained in use. Bleeding, purges, and blisters to draw out 'morbid matter' were standard remedies. Herbal and chemical medicines were sold by apothecaries without consultation with a licensed physician. Apothecaries far outnumbered doctors in European cities in 1800, and most persons consulted a doctor as a last resort. Perhaps because of the severity of standard treatments, homeopathic procedures (like cures like) were popular. Homeopathic remedies such as small doses of cinchona (quinine) or belladonna were far less toxic than many treatments in common use.[21]

The germ theory was not substantially developed until the second half of the nineteenth century, when the compound microscope was improved, the theory of spontaneous generation of microbes disproved, and techniques for isolation of microbes in laboratory cultures developed. The contagionists were ultimately vindicated, but in fact the miasmatic theories which led to sanitation programs to remove noxious substances probably reduced disease mortality more effectively than the quarantines of the early nineteenth century.

Thus European and Muslim medicine embodied similar ideas concerning epidemics derived from empirical observation, the common Judaeo-Christian–Islamic heritage, and from Galenic (Greek) medicine. By 1800 the two systems of thought had only begun to diverge. During the nineteenth century, medicine was to advance rapidly in European and in Muslim regions. In Tunisia, the mechanism of this advance must be studied not only in the context of the Industrial and Scientific Revolutions, but in the context of the colonial encounter that revolved around new commercial and political power struggles.

Chapter 1

Indigenous medicine against plague, 1780–1830

Today, walking up the hill on the main street of the old city of Tunis, one passes former Ottoman barracks, stately Arab villas closed off from the narrow lane by wooden gates, shops selling hand-woven carpets, perfumes, and inlaid metalware. The street is full of jostling, milling crowds, pressing their way to work or to shops. The Great Mosque, built in its present form in the ninth century by the Aghlabid rulers, faces a row of herb shops where medicines are sold. The shops are colorful, with jars of spices, herbs collected in the countryside, camphor, and imported metallic compounds. Turning to the right, one crosses to another busy street, Nahj al-Qasaba, or rue de la Kasbah, where, at number 101, the old *maristan* (hospital) of Tunis is located. Continuing up the street, one suddenly enters a main square around which is the Dar al-Bey, or bey's palace, built by Hamuda Bey al-Husayni (1782–1814) and now the site of the prime ministry. Across the square is the newer Muslim hospital, the Mustashfa Sadiqi, and at the top the Kasbah (citadel).

Two hundred years ago Tunisia was ruled from the Kasbah by the Husayni dynasty of beys,[1] who had become Arabized and who paid formal allegiance to the Ottoman sultan and ruled independently. Hamuda Bey presided over a prosperous territory which enjoyed a brisk trade with southern Europe, the Levant, and sub-Saharan Africa. Tunisia, located just 85 miles from Sicily, was at the center of the east–west and north–south long-distance trade routes, its port of La Goulette crowded with ships transporting wheat and olive oil to France, manufactured goods to Egypt and Syria, and business-minded pilgrims from the Maghrib and West Africa to Mecca. Its people were participating in international trade and travel and thus were subject to contagious diseases from outside.

Indigenous public health and medicine

Provisions for public health in the city of Tunis compared favorably with those in Mediterranean port cities of the eighteenth century. The city

14

was not considered exceptionally unhealthy by contemporary European travelers. Shaw, an English physician and traveler, recorded his impressions of the city in 1727:

The many Lakes and Marshes that surround this City, might probably render the situation of it less healthy, were not these Inconveniences in some Measure corrected by the great Quantity of Mastick, Myrtle, Rosemary, and other gummy and aromatic plants, that are daily used in the heating of their ovens and Bagnios,

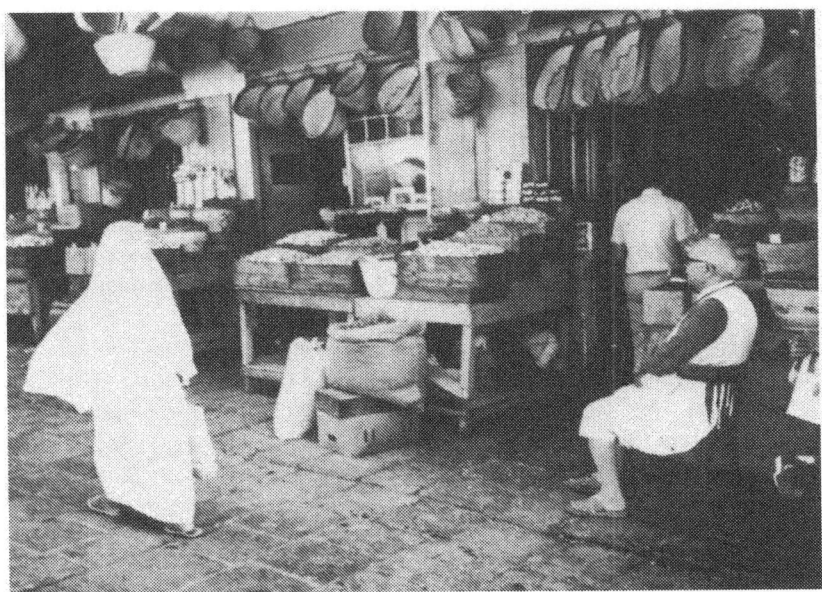

Fig. 1. Medicinal herb shops

and which frequently communicate to the air a sensible fragrance. The want of water is another complaint of the Tunisiens, who for the Brackiness of their well water and the scarcity of cisterns, are obliged to fetch a greater part of what they drink from Bardo, and other Places at eleven miles distance. If we accept This Inconvenience, no Place enjoys a greater Plenty of all the necessaries of Life.[2]

The problem of water supply was critical. Most houses had cisterns dug beneath them, where rainwater was collected. Families then drew their water from courtyard wells. But when rainfall was scarce, or during the summer months, water was often lacking. A water supply system had been constructed by Hamuda Bey's father, 'Ali Bey (1759–82), in the 1770s as one of his many public construction projects. He had renovated waqf-endowed water systems that had fallen into disrepair, and ordered the Ras Tabi'a spring connected to the Roman aqueduct, which was also repaired.

Water from the hot springs at the foot of Jabal Ahmar, eight miles from the capital, was brought to the Kasbah by means of a large underground pipeline constructed of masonry. This pipeline was fed by seven wells along its edges and branched out in the madina into underground canals along the streets. Twenty public fountains were supplied by this pipeline.[3]

'Ali Bey also renovated wells in the quarters of Bab Suwiqa and Bab Jazira. They were equipped with *na'ura*s (large water wheels) which drew water from newly constructed reservoirs. Irrigation systems in other areas were also expanded. Kairouan was provided with additional reservoirs for agricultural expansion.[4]

But since the masonry from which the pipelines were constructed was not regularly maintained, contamination of the private and public water supply systems was inevitable. Most household refuse was put into pits dug near each dwelling; from there, rainwater washed the refuse into large open-air drains (*khanduqs*) which led down the hill to the Lake of Tunis.[5]

The drains became like rivers in the wintertime when heavy rains fell. During the summer, inhabitants complained about the dust. The Lake of Tunis emitted sulfurous fumes from the decomposing matter in its shallow waters. Some eighteenth-century travelers considered the fumes a healthy disinfectant. Others felt the burning of aromatic plants helped purify the dangerous sulfurous air. Desfontaines (a doctor who was in Tunisia during the plague of 1784), for example, thought that burning aromatic plants helped purify the air polluted by the infected exhalations that rose from the banks of the lake and from the drains that collected the refuse of the 'enormous city'.[6]

During the eighteenth century the practice of burying the dead within city walls was discontinued. Because it was thought that epidemics spread by miasmas or bad air, cemeteries were moved outside the city walls. The largest Muslim cemetery was the Jalaz cemetery located on the hill of Sidi Bilhasan, the famous Shadhili shrine. The Catholic cemetery, which had been near Bab al-Bahr (Port of the Sea, now Porte de France), was also moved farther from the center of town.

In addition, there were certain provisions for personal hygiene, such as the *hammam* (public bath). The city had numerous hammams, some exclusively for women, others for men on some days, women on others.[7] The hammams and the hot mineral springs located in various regions of Tunisia were frequently used for the treatment of disease.[8]

The indigenous medical establishment functioned during this time as it had for centuries. In the city of Tunis the bey appointed an *amin al-atibba'* (chief of doctors) to issue licenses or certificates of competence to practice (*ijaza*s) and to direct the maristan. According to Louis Frank, a French doctor who practiced in Tunis in the early nineteenth century, there were at least twenty-five doctors licensed by the amin there.[9] The amin issued ijazas on the basis of the applicant's experience, sometimes certified by a document signed by witnesses. The ijazas followed a standard form. Fig. 2 shows one such license, issued in 1818 and renewed in 1855. (There are grammatical and orthographic errors.) It reads as follows:[10]

Praise be to God. Our certificate is hereby in the hand of our son, Muhammad b. Muhammad al-Kilani. We certify him to cure injuries and illnesses. We free his hand in that, and no other doctor may oppose him, according to custom. Greetings from the servant to his God.

[signed] Muhammad al-Hajj Hasuna bu 'Asida, amin al-atibba'

1234/1818

The renewal was written by a different hand and signed Muhammad bu 'Asida, presumably son of the former amin. The recipient, al-Kilani, later became amin himself (see Chapter 4), and his son worked as an orderly under the direction of the first French-educated Tunisian doctor.

The amin did not have authority over the few European doctors who practiced in Tunisia, but as Frank commented, it was well to stay on good terms with him because he could be useful and his enmity could expose one to difficulties.[11] Occasionally the amins were medical scholars; Ahmad Dihmani al-Qayrawani, who was amin al-atibba' during the late eighteenth century, prepared a work on syphilis using European source materials. He traveled to Cairo for further study and apparently died there about 1835.[12]

In addition, there were about 120 Muslim and Jewish barbers in Tunis who bled patients and sometimes scarified sore muscles and cauterized injuries.[13] There were herb sellers, bonesetters, eye doctors, midwives, and circumcisors. As elsewhere in North Africa, marabouts wrote out amulets. Holy shrines (also called marabouts) were thought to cure through the power of baraka conveyed by the saint buried within.

Since at least the early eighteenth century, however, the beys had patronized European doctors as their personal physicians. The bey's European physician and the amin al-atibba' apparently shared medical authority, at least in the role of coroner. The earliest reference to the parallel functions of the amin al-atibba' and the bey's personal physician is found in the eighteenth-century chronicle *Kitab al-bashi*: 'In 1754, a

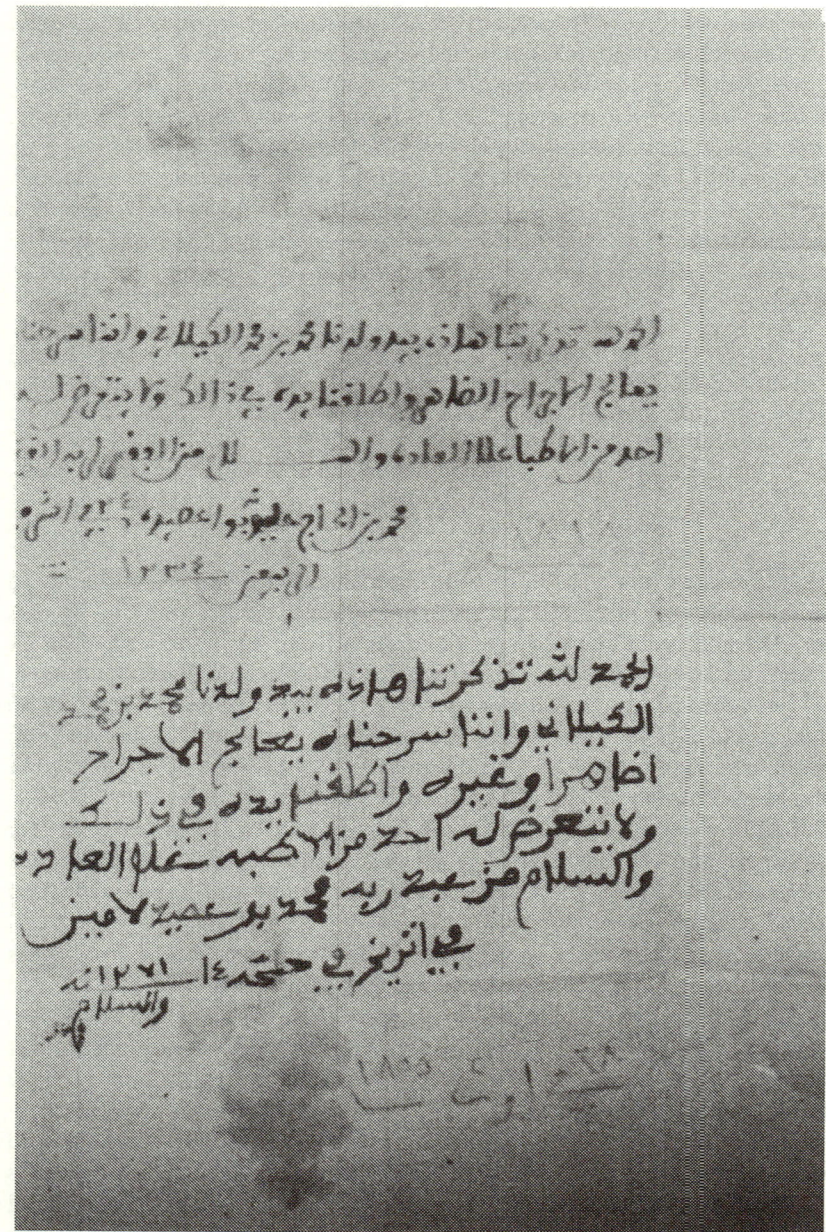

Fig. 2. Ijaza issued in 1818 to Muhammad b. Muhammad al-Kilani by Muhammad b. al-Hajj Hasuna bu 'Asida; renewed in 1855 by Muhammad bu 'Asida

son of 'Ali Bey was murdered by poisoning according to Muhammad al-Tabib al-Maghribi, amin al-atibba' and Yusuf al-Qurir, convert to Judaism from Christianity, doctor to the court of the capital....' The name of the former indicates that he was a Muslim, a doctor, and of Moroccan origin. Many of the doctors in Tunisia were from Morocco since people from there were believed to have special medical knowledge. The name of the latter was certainly Arabic for Joseph Curillo, who was of Italian, probably Livornese–Jewish, origin and was known to have practiced medicine in Tunisia, where he wrote several medical works. Thus, in the mid-eighteenth century, two medical authorities were relied upon – the Muslim chief of the doctor's order and the bey's European doctor.[14]

The beys used their personal doctors in commercial and diplomatic negotiations with Europeans. European doctors were more familiar than the bey with European protocol and diplomatic procedures and, having access to the bey for medical reasons, were able to play the role of mediator. Exemplifying this political–commercial–medical role was M. Pignon, a French doctor who practiced at court during the 1740s. Pignon was also president of the major French commercial company in Tunisia (the Compagnie Royale d'Afrique) and French consul at Tunis. A doctor with access to the inner court, he was in an ideal position to obtain and provide information on commercial and political matters to the bey, and presumably to his own company and government as well. Another doctor, Bruno Jourdan, was 'Ali Bey's personal physician in the 1770s. He was also active in commercial affairs and trade negotiations between Tunisia, Austria, Venice, and Tuscany. In recognition of his diplomatic efforts, Jourdan was appointed Austrian and Tuscan consul at Tunis. Hamuda Bey himself wrote the French consul to send him a good doctor from France.[15]

European doctors also practiced outside court. One, renamed Rajib, was a European convert to Islam.[16] He was to receive a dismal punishment during a plague outbreak he first diagnosed. Others, captured by privateers, were ships' doctors and practiced medicine while awaiting ransom. A few were travelers, such as Drs Frank and Desfontaines, in Tunis to learn about indigenous medical practices and remedies. Some military surgeons and doctors were occasionally hired by the bey. Dr Zehler of Strasburg accompanied Hamuda Bey's tax-collecting expedition for many years.[17]

The rulers of Tunis demonstrated their interest in European doctors from at least the early eighteenth century, and probably before. Through trade, diplomacy, and war, they learned of new scientific and medical ideas and sought to import technical advice and to add such clearly useful information to their own store of knowledge. They thought the Galenic–Islamic system was to be supplemented with the new discoveries and they seldom sponsored experimental research projects designed to test old ideas and uncover new theories and practices.

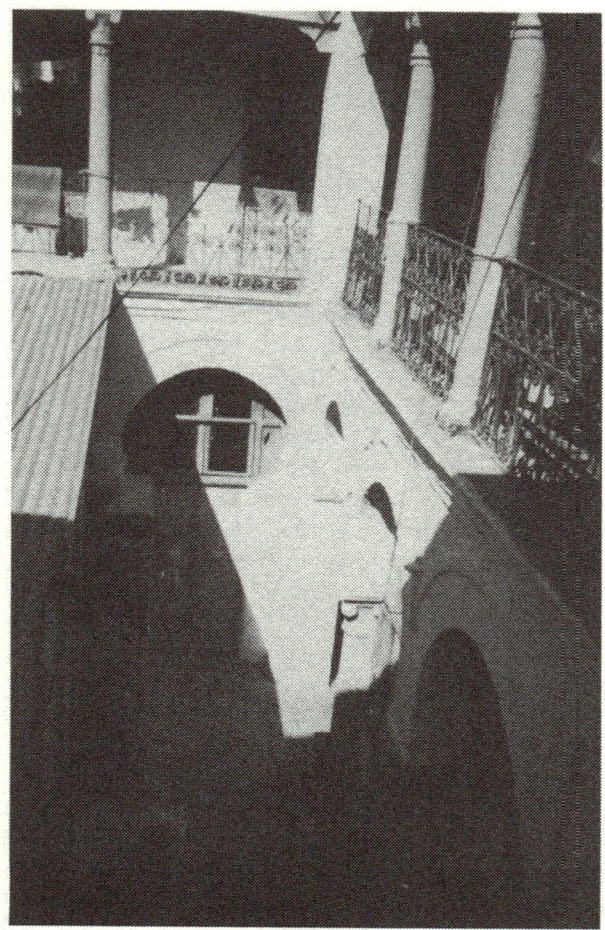

Fig. 3. Maristan of Tunis

In addition to their medical, political, and diplomatic advantages, European doctors perhaps conferred a certain prestige, rather like European fashions in clothing or furniture. The Ottoman sultans also liked to have a Jewish–Italian or Greek Orthodox doctor at court along with the Muslim chief of physicians, and this may have set the style for the beys. Benjamin Rush, the famous American physician, commented in 1793: 'It is remarkable that the effects of patronage, whether it be derived from titles or money, are as little influenced by success in the treatment of diseases as they are by talents.'[18] Yet despite the bey's patronage of European doctors, the indigenous medical structure continued to function until the 1860s independent of the bey's personal physicians.

Apparently as late as 1837, some Europeans in fact opted to work within the indigenous medical institutions. A letter preserved in the government archives at Tunis from the French consul to the *sahib al-taba‘* (keeper of the seal), Mustafa, requested employment in the maristan of Tunis for an unemployed French surgeon. A surgeon was not trained as a physician and no licence was presented. His previous experience, as stated in the letter, was with the *mahalla* (tax-collecting militia).[19] There is no reply to the request on record.

The maristan in which he sought work was founded in 1662, and from that time to 1879 was the only Muslim hospital in Tunis. It was founded by the ruler Hamuda Basha al-Muradi (1659−75), who set up a *waqf* (religious endowment) for the hospital funded by revenues from designated properties (see Appendix A).[20] The maristan was established in a two-story *funduq* (merchants' hotel) with twenty-four rooms, built around a central courtyard which opened from the *saqifa* (vestibule). The waqf revenues derived from inns, shops, public ovens, kilns, public baths, mills, water from certain springs, and rent from specified houses. The properties were located in various quarters of Tunis, Beja, Le Kef, Zaghouan, and Bizerte. The waqf document designated funds and provisions for a doctor, nurses, and servants. Salaries per day, in 1662, were:[21]

Amin al-atibba'   8 nasris, 4 loaves of bread per day, all the potions, herbs, oils, ointments, and bandages required, and a room in the maristan in which to sit

Supervisor   6 nasris, 4 loaves of bread

Cook   5 nasris, 2 loaves of bread

Overseer of expenses   4 nasris, 2 loaves of bread

Bawwab [doorman]   8 nasris, 4 loaves of bread (he was to stay in the maristan day and night)

The status of the doctor is suggested by the fact that he was paid no more than the doorman though he could presumably supplement his income with other consultations. The salaries were comparable with daily wages of the time; medicine was a craft like other occupations. The waqf document stated that the patients had the right to remain until cured, and there was to be no distinction between Arabs, Turks, or other (Muslim) foreigners. The hospital was intended for the sick and wounded of the army and navy and for the poor who had no shelter nor persons to care for them in the city.

In addition to the maristan, in 1775 a *takiya* (hospice) also began to provide for public welfare. Founded by the ruler, 'Ali Bey (1759–82), it was located at Dabdaba near the Kasbah, was built in the form of a large *madrasa* (school), and included a mosque, a kitchen, and eighteen rooms for the infirm. There was also a twelve-room building, located at Bab al-Bahr near the entrance to the city, for women with incurable diseases or mental disturbances. The main function of the takiya, however, was to supply food to the needy. It became known as the 'takiyat al-kuskusu' after the food served (couscous, a North African staple).[22] Each needy individual received about a half riyal's worth of food per day. In the 1820s, over 160 men and women were supported by the takiya.[23]

A large waqf endowment made by 'Aziza 'Uthmana (d. 1646), a daughter of 'Uthman Dey, of the Muradi dynasty (r. 1598–1610), funded both the maristan and the takiya in the early nineteenth century. The granddaughter of 'Aziza, Fatima, added to the principal of the endowment. 'Aziza 'Uthmana is remembered for her numerous charitable endowments which in the nineteenth century came to be centered on the maristan, supplementing or replacing Hamuda Basha al-Muradi's waqf. The maristan was often referred to as Mustashfa 'Aziza 'Uthmana ('Aziza 'Uthmana Hospital). Revenues came from crops of dates, olives, pomegranates, and sweet limes, and from shops, hammams, and rents on buildings. According to waqf accounts, salaries were allocated per month to trustees, the government head scribe or secretary, servants, and two doctors, one of whom was 'not needed' (see Fig. 4).[24]

The maristan continued in operation until 1879. Nearly all European travelers mentioned the maristan in their descriptions of the city. Most commented on its inadequacy. Count Filippi in 1829 claimed that the waqf funds for the hospital were being embezzled by the wakil, who was appointed by the bey.[25] Accounting was apparently rudimentary: there is only one receipt in the government archives of the maristan's records. It states that in 1252/1836, Ahmad al-Safi, wakil of the maristan, received 500 riyals from Hasan al-Sha'ar, instead of Bakar b. Jab'i, the former wakil.[26] In about 1850, a Dr Brandin wrote to Dr Bertherand in Algeria that there was but one hospital for the indigenous Arabs and Berbers of Tunis: 'It is so miserable and lacking in services that it should

	Riyals
Salary of *wakil* [trustee] and first notary, Si 'Ali Tamimi, and 10 guests of the Great Mosque and Bashir Ahmad Ibn Mahrus and his relatives	300
Salaries per month for administration:	
Second notary, Si Muhammad al-Sabi'	30
Third notary, Si Muhammad al-Sharif	30
Fourth notary, Si Hajj 'Uthman al-Sanusi	30
Fifth notary, Si al-Mukhtar al-Sharif	30
Shaykh Katib, Si al-Baji al-Mas'udi	300
Shaykh Si al-Hajj 'Uthman al-Shamigh	90
Si 'Ali b. al-Shaykh Bash Mufti Sidi Salih al-Nifi (and he does not take anything from it)	90
	600
Expenses for the maristan per month:	
First notary Si Muhammad al-Hashishi, the deputy, the doctor, the cook, and four servants	450
Salaries per month for administration:	
Second notary, Si al-Tahr Dakhil	45
Third notary, Si al-Kilani al-Qalibi	45
Fourth notary, Si al-Mukhtar al-Sharif	45
Second doctor, Si Isma'il, who is not needed	60
	195
Military maristans take what is necessary from medicines and materials for preparing the dead for burial from funds outside this account	
Expenses for the takiya per month:	
Wakil, first witness, Si Bilhasan, *imam* [prayer leader], *mufti* [legal authority], and expenses for debts	340.200
Expenses for the poor: 27 men	555
Expenses for the poor: 24 women	390
Upkeep for poor outside takiya	360
	1,645.200
Grand total	3,190.200

Fig. 4. Monthly budget of 'Aziza 'Uthmana Waqf

be considered an anticipated tomb rather than a place where pain can find alleviation.'[27]

Smaller waqf-supported maristans and takiyas functioned in Sfax, Sousse, and other cities.[28] The vast majority of the population, however, did not seek institutional care and sought assistance from relatives or local practitioners when afflicted with disease.

Owing to the threat of epidemic disease, the beys of Tunisia had, since the early eighteenth century, been accustomed to quarantine or refuse entry to ships from ports where it was known to exist. In 1722, for example, when cases of plague had been announced in Marseilles,

Husayn Bey (1705–25) refused admittance to all ships from the infected port and then added a twenty-day quarantine on all ships coming from France.[29] The authorities had established a small lazaret (quarantine station) on an island in the Lake of Tunis where goods were transferred while ships were waiting in quarantine.[30] When plague was announced in Algeria in 1755, desert caravans from Algeria were refused entry at the border, and in 1767, when a few cases of plague occurred in Tunisia, 'Ali Bey decided to remain within his palace and to deny customary public access to it.[31] The earliest record of the quarantine in the Tunisian archives, however, dates from the reign of Mahmud Bey (1813–14).[32]

Commercial–political disagreements resulting from quarantine policies could lead to war. In 1789 Hamuda Bey broke relations with Venice, a rival commercial center, over an incident in which Tunisian merchants had commissioned a Venetian ship to carry cargo from Alexandria to Tunis. Plague broke out on board, and the captain put in at Malta. There the quarantine officials ordered the cargo burned to destroy 'plague contagion'. The Tunisian merchants then asked the captain for compensation since they had put their property under his trust. The dispute led to a declaration of war on Venice, and the Tunisian corsair ships went to sea to seize compensation from Venetian ships. In reprisal, warships from Venice set sail and bombarded the city of La Goulette. The fleet then sailed to Sousse and Sfax, where they trained their cannons on the cities and fired upon them for days. Finally a cease-fire was arranged, terms were agreed upon, and regular commerce resumed.[33] Politics, commerce, and quarantines were inseparable in the eighteenth- and nineteenth-century Mediterranean economy.

Communal responses to plague, 1784–1820

In 1784, plague had not been seen in epidemic form for nearly eighty years. It must have seemed that the quarantine was working. But early in the year, plague struck again. The disease was apparently brought into Tunisia by passengers from a French ship carrying pilgrims returning from Mecca. The ship's voyage originated in Alexandria; on the way to Tunis, plague broke out among the passengers on board. Though it was illegal to land with plague cases on board, the captain avoided the quarantine authorities and docked his ship at La Goulette, where the passengers disembarked. The disease spread rapidly throughout Tunisia, immobilizing the capital city from the spring of 1784 until the summer of 1785, and was remembered as *al-waba' al-kabir* (the Great Epidemic).[34]

As the number of victims rose, all resources of the society were called upon to combat the epidemic. These included public health policies ordered by the bey, medical treatments based on existing medical theories, and religious precautions suggested by the '*ulama*' (religious scholars). Hamuda Bey does not seem to have isolated himself at the first news of the disease. But like his father, 'Ali Bey, he subsequently prevented his subjects from coming too close to him by means of a barricade which he installed in the audience room of the Bardo palace.[35] He then abolished the custom of hand kissing and did not receive letters unless they had been sprinkled with vinegar, thought to be a disinfectant. This last precaution was apparently adopted on the advice of European consuls. He also forbade burials within the city walls and ordered that graves be dug at least two meters deep so that the fumes from the decomposing corpses would not cause harmful miasmas, thought by some to cause plague.[36]

Apparently, the populace did not resent these protective measures. In 1724, Peyssonnel, the French doctor and traveler, had asked Muslims in Tunis about the quarantine. He was told that Tunisia owed its freedom from plague to it.[37] European visitors in Tunis during the epidemic of 1784–5 were nearly unanimous, however, in their reports of fatalism among the Muslim communities during the epidemic. In 1789, for example, Abbé Poiret published his account of his experiences:

The system of predestination so generally adopted by all the Mahometans, renders the Moors almost indifferent to whatever may befall them.... Amidst the great misfortunes, they make use of no other expression but this, God will have it so.... It is also to this comforting prepossession that they are indebted for that indifference with which they behold the plague exercising the greatest ravages among them. How often have I seen them, during this destructive contagion, wait for death without the least emotion, discharge all the duties of humanity to those who were infected, cleanse their ulcers, inter the dead, and without any precaution, put on the clothes of those who had perished by this cruel malady.[38]

In this vein, Père Vicheret, a priest in Tunis, recorded in his diary stories he had heard about houses in which all the inhabitants had died of the plague. One house was owned by the bey, who sold it to another family. They too died within a few days. It was sold again to another family. They too died within a few days. It was sold to another family, which also perished. In the course of the 1784–5 epidemic, the house was sold seventeen times. Vicheret added that there were other houses that were emptied five, six, eight times, adding to the profit of the bey.[39]

The actual motivation in such cases was evidently economic, the possibility of material loss outweighing the possible risk of plague. And many did not recognize the principle of contagion (transmission of the disease by contact with the infected persons or their possessions). In one instance, Hamuda Bey ordered that the clothes and possessions of the deceased be burned, on the advice of the consuls who remembered the practice from European public health procedures. Houses in which a plague victim had died were to be shut for several weeks. Hamuda also ordered that the itinerant sick be isolated in the *makhzan*s (storehouses) of the potters. People did not understand why these measures were taken as they 'saw no medical reason for them', and they strongly resented the destruction of property resulting from the bey's order. As the burnings continued, complaints abounded to the point of rioting. Some of the 'ulama' of the capital, believing reliance on God to be the best course of action, composed a poem in opposition to the bey's orders:

> The people of integrity and knowledge say:
> We entrust ourselves to the Merciful, the Creator
> The Creator and the Almighty
> None but He had the power of events
> We were ordered to recite a *dhikr* [recitation of sacred words] and an
> invocation
> He is what saves from an epidemic[40]

Nevertheless, the bey persisted in his order. When the protests increased, he took his case to the mufti and senior 'ulama' for adjudication. They ruled it was 'unfair to add to the misery of the people by ordering the burning of their clothes, as their duty was to surrender to the will of God'. This view was tempered with another statement, that the relatives of the deceased were 'widows and orphans of the dead and had the right to seek recompense for the destroyed property'. The 'ulama' were suggesting that the bey should provide compensatory funds to the relatives if he wished to continue his policies. In conclusion, the 'ulama' added that they 'saw the medical necessity for the order but felt that it caused too much hardship for the people'. For a time, the bey held his ground and the protests continued. After further correspondence with the *shaykh al-madina* (head official of Tunis), who disliked implementing the policy, the bey finally rescinded the order and the crisis ended.[41]

This new European-style preventive measure was not a success. The public, represented by the 'ulama', was able to exert its will upon the bey, who was in turn doing his best to fight the disease. The populace had its own medical concepts which did not call for destruction of property. Muslim medical traditions in the eighteenth century seemed at least as effective as their European counterparts so why go to such unpleasant lengths?

In Tunis books by Muslim religious and medical authorities enjoyed wide circulation and were kept on hand for home remedies and personal consultation. Among the more popular in the eighteenth and nineteenth centuries were the works of Yusuf al-Sanusi al-Hasani (d. 1486), Jalal al-Din al-Suyuti (d. 1505), and Da'ud al-Antaki (d. 1599). Al-Sanusi, in his *Mujarrabat al-dirbiy al-kabir* (*Experiences of the Great Dirbiy*), offered several talismans against plague: 'On a paper write the *basmala* [invocation], Almighty God, the Living, the Standing, the Judge, the Just, the Holy, then *Sura* [Chapter] 6, *Aya* [Verse] 122, and part of Sura 13, Aya 31, then this *khatm* [seal]: Ꮮ ᵩ |||| ⌗ ᵳ ⅏ ☆ then the name of the person it is for, followed by these letters:

Ꮮ Ꮮ Ꮮ Ꮮ ﺝ ⊃ ⊃ ﺡ ﺡ.'[42]

In his *Tibb al-nabiy* (*Medicine of the Prophet*), al-Suyuti suggested that plague came from contact with diseased persons, from spontaneous putrefaction, from meteorites, or from scarcity of rain, all of which could alter the humors, but that amulets against the spirits were accepted by the Prophet as a possible preservative.[43] In another work, *al-Rahma fi al-tibb wa al-hikma* (*Blessings of Medicine and Wisdom*), he provided lengthy *du'a*'s (invocations) similar to those of al-Sanusi. He also recommended a remedy of milk and urine of camel taken morning and evening or a portion of water in which a red hot iron had been plunged.[44] Al-Antaki, in his *Tadhkirat*, also thought plague was caused by atmospheric changes that could stir up the jinn. He wondered why some sources said that plague was a punishment for sin, others that it was martyrdom for believers, and still others that it was a result of an imbalance of humors. In a compromise solution, he concluded that plague was a punishment for hypocrites and infidels but that the most likely victim was one whose humors were not in balance. He then recommended bleeding the plague-stricken individual. The patient was to abstain from hot foods such as meat, which caused increased circulation of the blood, and was to eat cool foods such as fruits instead.

Aromatic substances such as bitter oranges, mint, vinegar, and apples placed in the sickroom were also beneficial. Burning of musk of amber or tar was similarly helpful. Ointments of bitter orange, sandalwood, vinegar, and camphor were rubbed on the body. A compound remedy to repel the poisons that accompanied the disease consisted of aromatic herbs, Armenian earth, gum arabic, amber, chalk, and rose water, taken in the form of a pill. A vomitive was also prescribed against the excess humor and the patient was cautioned to refrain from going to the baths.[45]

Often, collections of talismans were also kept in hand. One such collection, preserved in the manuscript collection of the Bibliothèque Nationale in Tunis, contains the following special *tasbih* (talisman or blessing): 'It is recommended that one say "there is no power and no strength save in God" one hundred times every morning and evening during time of epidemic... [or one can say] seven times, after each prayer, the names Mustafa, Murtada, his two sons and Fatima to extinguish the heat of the epidemic....'[46] Plague buboes were suppurated and pieces of alum with the words 'laghigh, baligh and talugh' written on them were placed on the abscesses. The words were names of the jinn believed to cause plague and alum was thought a repellent to them. Thus surgical and symptomatic remedies were combined with anti-jinn treatments.[47]

Dr Shaw, the English physician who visited Tunisia in the early eighteenth century, found this account of a preservative used against plague, issued by a marabout, Sidi Muhammad Zarruq: 'The life of all is in the hands of God and when his hour is come he will die. However, it pleases providence to preserve persons from plague who take each morning while the epidemic exists one or two pills composed of myrrh and syrup of grains of myrtle.'[48] Shaw learned that Muslim doctors suppurated plague buboes with leaves of opuntia steeped in water. In 1724 Peyssonnel, the Marseilles doctor, sent back to his sponsors in France medical information on Muslim treatments for plague in Tunisia. He reported that Muslim doctors suppurated the buboes with a scille or Spanish onion, or with butter mixed with honey.[49] Europeans were curious about Muslim methods in the wake of the Marseilles epidemic but as the decades passed with no further outbreaks, they gradually lost interest.

The majority of Europeans living in Tunisia during the 1784–5 epidemic were captives, imprisoned in Tunis by privateers, awaiting ransom by relatives or by their governments. More fortunate were the twenty or thirty merchants and consuls resident in Tunis. Throughout the Muslim Mediterranean, European residents of plague-stricken towns customarily retreated to their funduq, where they remained for the duration of the epidemic. Plague was nearly forgotten in their home cities and was a disease associated with foreign places; they could take refuge from it by avoiding local inhabitants. Plague had become a disease for non-Europeans or at least a disease to be found in 'the east', an unwholesome place. But the cause of plague was not suspected.

Merchants isolated themselves within the funduq for weeks and even months, until the cases of plague were no longer announced daily. Complicated rules to avoid contracting the disease were circulated by European consuls or priests at the outbreak of each epidemic and recalcitrant persons were often ordered by their consuls to shut themselves in. Once inside they took elaborate precautions to avoid contact with the outside. In Tunis the French merchants stayed in their funduq near Bab al-Bahr. Communications with the outside were accomplished through the aid of *piskeries*, natives of the city of Biskra in southeast Algeria, who worked in Tunis as street porters. The intermediaries purchased food and other provisions for the inhabitants and placed the provisions on long pincers that had been fumed with absinthe (wormwood). The items were then fumed and taken inside. Sacks of flour were particularly suspect (justifiably so since rat fleas could harbor there) and were aired before use.

During the 1784 epidemic the local priest, Père Vicheret, issued a set of procedures to follow to minimize the danger of contracting plague. He recommended eating rice, vegetables, and herbs, and no meat. He thought that a glass of wine did no harm and that bread carried no miasmas.[50] He advised against buying cloth of wool or cotton unless absolutely necessary and ordered that these items be sprinkled with fresh water to extinguish the miasmas. He also recommended the use of vinegar, quinine, camphor, absinthe from the mountains of Tunisia, or other strongly aromatic herbs. Vicheret's recommendations resembled those of al-Antaki in the use of aromatic herbs and special foods. The avoidance of textiles was probably a result of empirical observation that made textiles themselves suspect. We now know infected fleas are easily transported in bolts of cloth. No one then understood that the disease was spread by fleas, although in Tunis there was a Muslim saying that plague was around during spring, extinguished in the heat of summer, then back in autumn 'like the fleas'.[51] Astral influences were widely suspect as causative agents in disease spread by Europeans and Muslims. In Tunis in 1785 a Dutch vice-consul 'confirmed' to Père Vicheret that plague 'crossed' with the moon.[52]

In 1784 none of the twenty or thirty shut-ins perished whereas about 140 of the several hundred European captives who were kept in unsanitary prisons died. But the merchants' self-imposed sanitary cordon may not have saved them because rats and fleas could have crossed the barriers. In fact, during the 1705 epidemic several Europeans perished from plague within their funduq. And in 1700, during a plague outbreak in Tunis, a Capuchin missionary priest heard confessions of plague victims within the funduq, from across a barrier. Despite the precautions, the priest caught the disease and died.[53]

During the plague the two communities viewed one another with mutual distrust. In his diary Père Vicheret recorded instances of hostility directed against Europeans by Muslims. The phrase 'May you all die [of the plague]' ('In challa todos morir' in Ladino, the lingua franca of the time) was called out to passing European funeral processions.[54] Desfontaines, the French doctor who had been in Tunisia during the 1784 epidemic, reported that in La Calle in western Algeria, the Nahad tribe, which had been decimated by plague, was irritated by the sight of the Christians enclosed in their funduq trying to escape the scourge. By burying their dead near the walls and throwing rags dipped in suppurating buboes over the walls,[55] the Muslims tried to introduce the disease among the Christians, indicating their belief in contagion and their resentment of the European presence.

Abbé Poiret, in turn, wondered at the 'calm' of the Muslims and their callousness during the 1784–5 plague:

Whoever, for example, newly landed upon these coasts, should advance towards the infected tents, whoever should have seen, as I, the father of a family distribute without a tear, to his wives and children the cloth which was to wrap up their bodies after death, and the latter receive it with a stoic tranquility, would undoubtedly imagine himself transported into a society of philosophers; especially if he should be present at the festivals, dances, and public displays of joy which they exhibit amidst the ravages of the plague.[56]

Other reports, in contrast, indicate that it was the Muslim communities who resented Europeans' public displays of joy during plague outbreaks. On one occasion, during a recurrence of plague in July 1794, French merchants were again enclosed within their funduq. There they were enthusiastically celebrating Bastille Day when the bey lost his temper. A consular letter of 1794 reported: 'Music and dancing and the most unrestrained licentiousness followed this dinner. The indignation of the bey was at its height. He stated that it was revolting that while the plague desolated his kingdom and there was not a family in Tunis that did not weep for a member, foreigners welcome in his regions had the courage publicly to rejoice.'[57] A month later Mustafa Khuja, the bey's prime minister, wrote to complain to the French consul: 'The conduct of the French is not satisfactory. They are firing shells on neighboring houses to the great alarm of their inhabitants, most of whom are occupied with their dead and dying following the plague which has devastated our capital. The noisy joy of the French seems out of place to the unhappy inhabitants and is a striking contrast to the public calm.'[58]

But all were ultimately forced to submit to the ravages of the disease. The epidemic of 1784–5 lasted for eighteen months. Those who survived estimated that one-sixth to one-third of the Tunisian population perished.[59] After the epidemic, ships were again issued clean bills of health (patents) and normal commerce resumed.

Plague, however, lingered in endemic form (constantly present, with low morbidity) in the 1790s. Ships departing from Tunisian ports occasionally carried patents indicating plague in Tunis. Incoming ships were usually admitted without hindrance since plague was then absent from most regions of the Mediterranean. The French merchants occasionally retreated to their funduq for safety but in general business went on as usual.

After a lapse of two decades, plague returned to Tunisia in epidemic form in 1818. Again, the communal responses reflect concern over the best means of prevention, a mystery yet to be solved. The disease again arrived on a ship returning from Mecca via Alexandria (or, some said, on a plague-infected ship from Istanbul that landed at Sousse). Rajib, the European doctor mentioned above who had converted to Islam from Christianity, was the first to diagnose plague. Enraged by the news, the bey had him bastinadoed and thrown into prison. Doctors in European cities received similar treatment when they announced the presence of plague. But while other doctors hesitated to diagnose the disease, plague spread throughout Tunis. European merchants as usual returned to their funduq and the bey reluctantly ordered sanitary cordons to be set up. A year later the epidemic began a second onslaught, during which time the French remained ensconced within their funduq. It lasted until July 1820.[60]

The sanitary cordons were apparently more strictly applied than during the earlier epidemic. Many of the city's inhabitants resented the blockades restricting traffic because, according to some interpretations of Islamic law, such preventive measures were not allowed.

Bin Diyaf, the famous chronicler, who was then fifteen years old, recorded that people in Tunis were divided into two groups. One group 'saw prevention in abstaining from mixing, by what is known as quarantine'. The other group 'did not see the usefulness of prevention except in surrender to the will of God'. The first group, which was proquarantine, was led by the prominent Hanafi *shaykh* (master) 'Abd Allah b. Muhammad b. Muhammad b. Muhammad Bayram III, who cited two well-known hadiths in support of his position: 'no contagion, no evil omen' and 'flee the leper as you flee the lion'. These hadiths call upon Muslims to reject superstition and to take action against potential danger. Bin Diyaf noted that the essence of 'no contagion' meant in context to reject the superstitious idea of contagion or infection while taking action against the actuality which experience had proven dangerous. He added that since one died at his appointed hour even if he took precaution, God's will would still be done. So why not take action?[61]

The second group was headed by the *katib* (scribe) Abu 'Abd Allah Muhammad Sulayman b. al-Mana'i, who cited the example of Abu 'Ubayda 'Amr b. al-Jarah. In 640, Abu 'Ubayda had opposed 'Umar b. al-Khattab when the latter refused to send his troops into plague-stricken

Syria. This group preferred holding an invocation as the surest defense against the disease. The following is an excerpt from a poem composed in support of this second position. It was prepared from the treasuries of invocations from the path of Shadhili, founder of the famous Sufi order:

> Oh, lord, how excellent a refuge are you.
>> Restore us to health and cure us for you are the cure.
> This plague is like the burning fire.
>> The hearts of the people are purified.
> How many people's livers are burst open.
>> The eagle sends away sorrow and joy.
> God is angry with our sins.
>> He punishes the enemies when they are disobedient.[62]

Supplication to the Almighty was of course the intent of the invocation, but the idea, familiar to Europeans, of plague as a punishment for sin was also expressed in the invocation.

The son and successor of the reigning bey, Husayn, was a partisan of the group favoring reliance on providence. During the 1818 epidemic 'he rallied against the officials of the quarantine and went around the streets and impasses of the capital where there were many sick, and went through the impoverished and severely stricken Jewish quarter saying "there is no flight from destiny"'. Bin Diyaf added that his actions 'strengthened the hearts of the inhabitants of the city'.[63]

The majority of those who took precautions were spared, according to Bin Diyaf, but he observed that all those who were saved believed it was the result of the act of God. He added that this validated the viewpoint of 'Umar b. al-Khattab.[64]

While people worried over quarantining, the disease waned and then spread again. Curative methods tried in 1784–5 by Muslims and Europeans remained in use and need not be repeated here. As before, despite claims of practitioners, no medical remedy proved reliable. Finally, in 1820, with the quarantine dispute unsettled, the disease vanished from Tunisia. It was to be the last plague epidemic to date to strike the region.

Social and economic consequences of plague, 1780–1830

During each plague epidemic, the Muslim and European communities of Tunis relied upon similar but inadequate medical concepts that resulted in uncertainty and confusion. In general, while familiar with the concepts of contagion and quarantine, Muslims were somewhat more reluctant to seek salvation in flight or self-isolation than Europeans. According to Bin Diyaf, however, the majority had in 1818 opted for the 'quarantine party' and were saved, presumably by self-isolation. Europeans, on the other hand, often relied on amulets and sometimes eschewed defensive measures such as quarantining, but at least in Tunis, those who could were required by their consuls to follow the carefully enforced and self-imposed house quarantine. But curiously when the antiquarantine Husayn became bey in 1824, he began to issue numerous quarantine orders which are still preserved in the goverment archives. Perhaps his idealism diminished when confronted with the responsibilities of state.

During the dispute of the burning of contaminated property, the 'ulama' mediated between the people and the bey, being accepted by both as sources of knowledge and wisdom. Aside from this incident, there was little evidence of social destabilization. The epidemics did reveal latent hostility between the Muslim and European communities but it was easily contained and the bey retained his authority. Most sectors of the economy also proved resilient, at least in the last decades of the eighteenth century.

Regular trade and commerce were, along with agriculture, the mainstay of the Tunisian economy. The extent of the cross-Mediterranean trade is reflected in the fact that just under half of all ships landing at Marseilles from North Africa in the 1790s came from Tunis, then called the Shanghai of the Mediterranean.[65] Trans-Saharan caravans brought slaves, gold dust, gum Arabic, and ostrich feathers for sale in Tunis or for export to other Mediterranean ports. Grain, olive oil, vegetables, soap, wool, sponges, and coral obtained off the north coast of Tunisia found ready buyers in European markets, and the red felt caps (*shashiyas*) manufactured in Tunisia were sold around the Mediterranean. In addition, privateering ships, often outfitted by the ruler or merchant elite, pillaged the coasts and ships of non-tribute-paying states such as Sardinia, Sicily, and the smaller islands.

Trade and privateering were important sources of revenue to the ruler, who sold export permits, collected customs duties, taxed booty, mediated ransom payments, regulated all ship arrivals and departures, and sold produce from his own estates on the international market. Throughout the eighteenth century, North Africa was regarded as the granary of southern Europe. Prices for wheat and olive oil rose steadily during the latter half of the century to the advantage of Tunisian cultivators. Tunisia did not rely entirely on export of raw materials at the time, as the export of shashiyas amounted to a substantial proportion of the incoming profits.[66]

Tunisia had maintained trade agreements with European states since at least the twelfth century. These had been negotiated and renegotiated over the centuries according to the political fortunes of the respective governments. In the mid-eighteenth century, the Husayni beys were consolidating their power and took steps to protect Tunisian merchants. Hamuda's father, 'Ali Bey (1759–82), had stopped the abusive practice of forced sale to the government of crops before harvest time at fixed (low) prices. Following the French Revolution and collapse of the monarchy in 1789, Hamuda Bey and his minister, Yusuf Sahib al-Taba', announced that existing trade agreements with France were canceled. The government then began selling export permits only to Tunisians, who were also exempt from export fees on grain, olive oil, and certain other products, giving them an advantage over European merchants.[67] Further, when the Tunisian merchant fleet was in port, no other armed ship of a foreign nation was allowed to enter. Since many merchant ships were armed, this policy favored Tunisian commerce. In 1792 Hamuda forbade Europeans from purchasing directly from local producers; henceforth all middlemen were to be indigenous Muslims. Tunisian Jews were restricted from internal domestic trade, but were allowed to participate without hindrance in international commerce.[68] These policies were successful in expanding Tunisian commerce. In 1780 French merchants owned four out of five ships transporting cargo to Marseilles. By 1806 there were 150 Tunisian, six French, and two Venetian merchants operating in Tunis. According to a French consular letter of 1808, the policies of Hamuda Bey and Yusuf Sahib al-Taba' had resulted in the concentration of three-fourths of the international trade in the hands of Tunisian merchants.[69]

As a result of this trade and the 10 to 30 percent of cultivator's income taxed annually, the government and several elite families had accumulated substantial fortunes by the beginning of the nineteenth century.

Tunisia in this era seemed embarked on a promising course; according to *Kitab al-bashi*, an eighteenth-century chronicle written in Tunis by a court official, Hamuda Ibn 'Abd al-'Aziz, the population was growing, building programs abounded, agriculture was thriving, and the economy was, at least for the elite, prosperous.[70]

Lucette Valensi has suggested that the epidemic may have been the major factor in the near-total reversal of prosperity in Tunisia after the turn of the century. According to her findings, the amount of land under cultivation in the region around Tunis decreased in the late 1780s and 1790s. In Beja land under cultivation seems to have remained constant in the 1780s and 1790s. Valensi comments: 'In fact, it was plague which was paralyzing rural activity and which, without having ceased, was exercising prolonged effects on agriculture. If the situation did not restabilize, it was without doubt a result of a new appearance of the epidemic that lasted until the end of the eighteenth century.'[71]

In contrast, available commercial records from the era seem to indicate continued prosperity. Masson, in his authoritative history of the Compagnie Royale d'Afrique, assembled trade statistics that seem to indicate peak years in Tunisia just following the epidemic:[72]

Value of imports from Tunis (primarily wheat and olive oil), and excluding coral and wool

Year	Value (livres)
1785	2,882,000
1786	2,745,000
1788	4,213,000
1789	3,762,000

The rapid increase in total trade is seen in the Chamber of Commerce records pertaining to trade with Tunisia:[73]

Year	Exports to Tunis (livres)	Imports from Tunis (livres)
1776–1780	3,804,000	4,246,000
1781–1785	3,693,000	10,747,000
1786–1789	3,879,000	14,308,000

The balance of payments was consistently in favor of Tunisia. On the increase in trade during the plague years, Masson remarked:

From the statistics prepared by the Chamber of Commerce, the exchanges of this port with Tunis, which had never exceeded 1,500,000 livres before 1770, and which until 1776, had reached 2,000,000 but once, nearly always exceeded this sum during the subsequent years, except during the American Revolutionary War. Many times, the figure of 3,000,000 was exceeded. Finally, in spite of a terrible plague which carried off, they say, 100,000 inhabitants of Tunis itself, the exchanges were from 4 to 6,000,000 livres.[74]

The French consul at Tunis attributed the increase in the export of wheat in the late 1780s to 'the simultaneous poor harvests in Europe and the abundance of crops in the kingdom of Tunis...[This had] led a throng of ships to the port of Tunis which in less than four years, had become the most rich and commercially active of the Levant.'

Such information is difficult to reconcile with the hypothesis that lack of manpower from population decrease caused agricultural production to fall sharply. If there had been threat of famine domestically, the bey would have been expected to forbid export of grain, but this did not occur.

There were, to be sure, indications of the severity of the epidemics. Perhaps because of exposure to fleas, an exceptionally large number of weavers, mat makers, and shashiya manufacturers perished. Before the epidemic the price of shashiyas was stabilized at 24 to 25 livres per dozen. Afterward the price rose sharply to 33 and 36 livres per dozen, attributable by contemporaries to the effects of the epidemic. But it is significant that the high-quality wool imported from France and Italy for use by the shashiya makers did not decline in quantity in 1783, 1784, or 1785 so the increase may have been temporary as new workers were trained, or it may have resulted from causes not related to plague.[75]

Furthermore, there is little indication of political weakness at the end of the century that can be clearly linked to the epidemics. Eighteenth-century Tunisia seems to have been resilient enough to absorb the shock of the devastation. Population levels had been increasing in the second half of the century and may have absorbed the heavy losses from plague. Perhaps inhabitants of the cities fled to the countryside and found seasonal work harvesting the annual crops, thus replacing those who had perished. The successes of the wheat crops in most regions of Tunisia in the second half of the 1780s suggest that plague cannot automatically be assumed to cause great and immediate economic loss even in labor-intensive agriculture.

The outbreaks of endemic plague that recurred in the 1790s in specific areas of the capital city and elsewhere were certainly a menace to daily life. Valensi has suggested that this period of plague caused a 'slow erosion of the population'. But according to Masson, French commerce with Tunisia increased markedly at the end of the century. Even the French Revolution did not impede regular trade: in 1792, for example, there were 79 merchant ships that sailed from Marseilles bound for Tunis. Tunisians were consuming more and the ships carried sugar, coffee, hardware, fabrics, spices, and drugs from Marseilles. In return, the ships brought oil, woolens, wheat, leather, beeswax, dates, beans, chickpeas, barley, and millet from Tunis, Sfax, and Sousse.[76]

By the second decade of the nineteenth century, however, the economic boom had come to an end. By 1810 there were signs of a recession.[77] In a French consular letter of that year commercial exchanges were reported reduced to pre-1776 levels after three decades of steadily increasing trade. The consul mentioned the plague of 1784 which had carried off a 'third' of the population as one possible cause but considered the restrictive policies of the beylical government primarily responsible for the recession.[78] In fact, however, international commerce relationships harmful to Tunisia were developing in a new political balance of power.

The Mediterranean trade which had been jointly pursued by European and Tunisian merchants experienced a significant transformation. Expanding European commercial interests were now able to dominate external trade in Tunisia and elsewhere. Thus the technological and scientific innovations of the Industrial Revolution, the political reorganizations generated by the French Revolution, and the subsequent release of entrepreneurial energies resulted in a new ability to impose terms on non-European regions.

At the same time, agriculture in Tunis was severely affected by a long drought during the first years of the nineteenth century. In the second decade international prices of grain and olive oil began to fall, largely as a result of the restabilization of agriculture following the Napoleonic Wars and the European famines of 1816 and 1817. By 1820 agricultural revenues had dropped by 12 to 40 percent of pre-1815 figures for the Tunisian government. Furthermore, manufactures produced in Marseilles had begun to compete with locally produced handmade merchandise to the disadvantage of indigenous artisans, especially after shashiya manufacture was introduced in southern France.[79]

After the Battle of Waterloo in 1815 European powers could direct their military might to other less urgent threats such as privateering ships from Morocco, Algeria, and Tunisia. For centuries, European and North African ships had raided one another. In the eighteenth century, with the growth of regular commerce, privateering declined. Only the smaller states such as Tunisia and islands such as Sicily, Sardinia, and Malta attacked each other. At the turn of the century, about 1500 captives were being held in Tunis. The bey himself invested in privateering enterprises and took a large commission for arranging ransom.[80] Now, with commercial exchanges multiplying, European powers were anxious to suppress the practice entirely.

In 1816, an English flotilla put in at the port of Tunis and convinced the bey to free all captives taken by privateers. In 1817, the American navy made a show of strength against the beylical government. In 1818 European powers meeting in Aix-la-Chapelle declared privateering detrimental to commerce and vowed to extinguish it. In 1819, French and English navies forced their terms upon the unwilling bey. Another source of revenue was lost at a time determined by European interests.[81]

The plague of 1818–20 was an event that, in people's memories, marked the end of an era dividing the past into good and bad times. In

Bin Diyaf's words, 'it was the first of many disasters to befall Tunisia after the death of Hamuda Bey, because it reduced the people of Tunisia by half and most of the cultivable land remained uncultivated'.[82] This demographic estimate is greatly exaggerated; extrapolating from mortality rates of Jewish residents of Tunis, perhaps a fifth of the population perished.[83] The epidemic was, however, far more visible to contemporaries than the changing military, political, and commercial balance of power. Thus, unlike the earlier epidemic of 1784–5, the 1818–20 plague occurred in a context of economic recession and its mortality seemed at least to cause the decline. Immediately after the epidemic, Tunisia's political fortunes worsened.

In 1824 a new trade treaty was presented to the bey by the French consul. Backed by a division of the French navy that had brought him to La Goulette, the representative of the French government was pressing for a new, more favorable commercial arrangement. In despair, Husayn Bey rediscovered his links with the Ottoman Empire and requested military aid from the sultan. But the Ottomans were pre-occupied with the Greek War of Independence and could send no support. The Ottoman defeat at Navarino in 1827, in which the Tunisian fleet was lost, once again demonstrated the strength of European military power. The relative military equality which had existed in the eighteenth century between Ottoman and European forces had been eroded. The 1824 treaty further solidified European economic interests while worsening Tunisia's already unfavorable balance of trade.[84] Moreover, while export profits declined, the desire for European manufactured goods within Tunisia increased. Competition from Syria and prohibitive tariffs in England and France further hurt the Tunisian textile industries. The drop in profits ruined many Tunisian commercial families and impoverished both the agricultural producers and the government. According to figures assembled by Mohammed Cherif, imports to Tunisia increased from 3.94 million francs in 1816 to 7.88 million in 1826–9 (annual average), an increase of 100 percent. Exports, however, increased from 4.61 million francs in 1816 to 6.76 million in 1826–9 (annual average), an increase of only 46 percent. These figures represent only legal trade; much more was actually exported illegally, including precious jewels. Much undeclared Tunisian money was exported, especially in specie. Of greater significance is the fact that exports included far fewer manufactured goods at the end of this period, indicating a decline in shashiya manufacture and in other domestic industries.[85]

European merchant houses established in Tunisia began loaning money at usurious rates to members of the elite who wished to purchase goods from abroad. Following near-bankruptcy in 1824 the government ordered the debasing of the currency. Inflation followed and since the intrinsic worth of the debased currency was less than its face value, it was not accepted for the purchase of imports. The non-debased silver currency of Tunisia flowed into the hands of European merchants, who became the sole possessors of exchangeable stable currency. By 1828 the government was indebted to local European merchants to the extent that the vice-consul of France accompanied the mahalla since part of the tax was consigned in advance to pay the debts.[86] Most of the rural populace was affected by the devaluation, being forced to accept the new currency for agricultural produce and then to purchase other products at inflated prices.

The economic decline cannot easily be ascribed to the epidemics. In time of prosperity, the plague had caused little immediate shock despite the population loss.[87] When the international context had dramatically shifted to the detriment of Tunisia, a second epidemic seemed to symbolize the beginning of hard times, at least in people's memories.

In 1820 there was little evidence that Europeans could better deal with plague than could Muslims. But the Muslim beys were anxious to adopt those remedies available to them that were derived from any source, whether from Muslim or European medical knowledge. Encounters between Muslim and European doctors took place on approximately equal terms. Public health measures such as quarantining of ships were, in popular expectation, responsibilities of the bey, who was personally charged with protection of his territories. When, however, a disease hitherto unknown in Tunisia struck in the mid-nineteenth century, new commercial patterns and political relationships called for a different approach to public health policies. Medical perceptions in subsequent decades were to change in accord with new scientific advances and, more importantly, with a new colonial power structure imposed upon the populace. In the following chapters, social responses to epidemics that occurred during the mid-nineteenth century reveal significant changes in the segments of the population which were most active in medical decision-making.

39

Chapter 2

Cholera in an age of European economic expansion, 1830–58

In 1830 France occupied Algiers and in the same year forced a new commercial treaty on the bey of Tunis. This treaty reinforced the ban on privateering and furthered the internationalization of the Tunisian economy. Under its provisions European governments with interests in Tunisia could establish consulates anywhere in the country regardless of the bey's wishes, government monopolies on indigenous industries were abolished, and European merchants were free to trade directly with Tunisian subjects, eliminating the necessity of purchasing export permits from the Tunisian government while European consuls retained the right to judge their own nationals. The treaty effectively nullified the advantages of Hamuda Bey's commercial policies that had stimulated and protected indigenous commerce during his reign. Furthermore, certain provisions in the treaty made France a 'special commercial partner' to the bey on highly advantageous terms to France, and rival Italian and English entrepreneurs were eager to join in such a partnership.[1]

During this era of European commercial expansion, relationships between European and Tunisian authorities changed not only in political and economic spheres but in institutions of medicine and public health. In the eighteenth century, the beys had complete control over quarantining but by the 1830s, European consuls assumed management. This was a new trend of shifting responsibilities from Muslim to European hands. Later in the century European colonial historians were to claim that their consuls had to step in to guide Tunisia in quarantine procedures because of the beys' heedlessness in the face of epidemic diseases. In reality, as is seen below, it was the beys' firmness with regard to quarantining that elicited the consuls' interest in taking over quarantine management. Quarantines interfered with business and business was increasingly conducted along guidelines set forth by European political backers.

At times the beys of Tunisia were more interested in enforcing firm quarantines than the European consuls, who objected to the interference in the flow of commerce. Husayn Bey (1824–35), who as prince and heir apparent had condemned the quarantine officials during the 1818–20 plague, emphatically enforced quarantine regulations when he became bey. In a letter to the French consul written in 1828 (see Appendix B), Husayn defended the quarantine to the consul, who wanted it suspended. He said that the quarantine was necessary to protect his people from outbreaks of disease spreading in various ports of the Mediterranean and that exceptions could not be made for some and not for others.[2] In a postscript, Husayn added that he believed the ten-day quarantine would not protect anyone in and of itself but he was obliged to try.[3]

In 1831 Husayn extended the quarantine to twenty days as a new disease, cholera, was spreading throughout the Mediterranean. He also sent a notice to the European consuls in Tunis announcing that all ships with patents stating 'disease present' were to return to a 'Christian port' to be quarantined, after which they would be admitted to Tunisia.[4]

Though these measures were similar to those taken in other Mediterranean ports, European shippers, who resented the bey's control over their affairs, considered them intolerable. Merchants and consuls were suspicious of quarantines because they considered them a tactic used to hurt their commercial interests. And in the early nineteenth century there was considerable controversy among European doctors as to whether diseases such as plague and cholera were in fact contagious. The quarantines caused critical delays and inconveniences and were resented by *laissez-faire* trade advocates as excess governmental interference. Expanded shipping magnified the issue of quarantining until it became a political problem. Complaints against the bey's seemingly arbitrary policies were regularly made from Tunis. In 1835 French merchants wrote to the Marseilles Chamber of Commerce:

At the news of the invasion of *cholera morbus* in Marseilles, the Bey, counseled by the foreign functionaries who look for concessions to ruin our commerce, has taken the inconceivable measure of refusing all incoming ships from our port. One cannot even receive packages. Captains Audiffren [?], Guirard and many others have been sent to Malta to do a quarantine of twenty one days and to have their letters purified. Thus, we remain without news of our families.... All business is suspended, and all orders cancelled.[5]

The bey's personal administration of quarantine was no longer acceptable to the Europeans and they were influential enough to insist that the matter be taken out of his hands. Rivalries among the merchants resulted in the assignment of the quarantine administration to the body of European consuls.

In 1835 Husayn's successor, Mustafa Bey (1835–7), called the consuls to his palace in the Kasbah to discuss the formation of a Sanitary

Council.[6] After deliberation they formed the first authorized European-run agency in Tunisia, but it had advisory powers only. It was to meet once a week for discussion and to advise the bey on public health matters that concerned Tunisia. The consuls hoped this would limit the possibility of favoring the ships of one nation at the expense of another. The meetings were taken very seriously; a secretary was appointed to take minutes, and the records of the council were carefully preserved. The council met for fifty years and the records became voluminous. Because of the unique information they supply, these records form a major source for this study.[7]

During the first decade of the council's existence, Italian was its lingua franca, though Arabic was used in correspondence with indigenous officials. In the 1850s French began to predominate as France's interests in Tunisia increased. The duties of the council were outlined during its first meeting on 19 November 1835.[8] The Sanitary Council took responsibility for all measures regarding ships arriving from abroad, while the governor of La Goulette (the only Muslim on the council) was charged with seeing to the fulfillment of the quarantine by all Tunisian ships. The council subsequently issued detailed regulations outlining the number of days of quarantine, the goods which were suspect under various circumstances, and the procedures for carrying out the quarantine.[9] Procedures were later coordinated with practices of other ports where similar councils functioned and were further standardized with the regulations issued at the International Congresses on Quarantine held in Paris in 1851, Istanbul in 1861, and Vienna in 1874.

Tunisia was thus brought into the Mediterranean commercial world much more intensively than had been the case in the eighteenth century. The rapidly growing commerce was important enough for its European representatives to be able to impose their policies with the sanction of the bey, who had little choice in the matter. In this fashion, the threat of cholera epidemic became an effective stimulus for the penetration of Europeans into the administrative apparatus of the beylical goverment. Even internal matters such as public health generated attention in places as far away as London and Paris. When a few cases of cholera occurred in the remote southern area of Tunisia, the British consular office hastily contacted the Foreign Office in London:

It is to be greatly feared that [Tunis] shall not escape, for the inhabitants of that part of the Regency [of Tunis] being chiefly Bedouins are not under much control.... If the malady should unhappily reach the town of Tunis, the consequences are to be apprehended to be dreadful among the lower classes of the inhabitants, particularly amongst the Jews living in the most miserable and filthy state. The medical aid is also very difficult.[10]

This consular report referred to the fact that the Bedouins were not likely to be controlled by a sanitary cordon. If cholera in fact spread to the capital, 'Europeans and their commerce would be threatened'. The European merchants and consuls were acutely aware of the danger posed by the disease itself and by urban rioting, which had resulted from cholera outbreaks in many European cities.[11] Fortunately, however, the disease did not spread northward but remained localized in the southern region. Tunisia had escaped the pandemic of the early 1830s and was one of the few regions with major ports to do so. Libya and Algeria were affected by the pandemic, as were the southern regions of Italy and France.[12]

Convinced of the effectiveness of quarantine, the Sanitary Council continued to meet and Tunisia remained cholera-free. The council took all the credit for this piece of good fortune; it proudly announced to Ahmad Bey in 1845, ten years after its inception:

In the year 1835, when the contagious sickness was afflicting a good part of the continent of Europe and of Africa, His Highness, the Basha Bey, the magnificent predecessor and father of Your Highness, with the voluntary agreement of the representatives of the foreign states, instituted a Council of Public Health, and entrusted to them its very important administration.... By means of the diligent and careful service of the employees and the rigorous precautions put into use by the Council of Public Health, the interior regions of the Regency are today in a state unharmed in any way by contagion.[13]

The Sanitary Council continued to issue quarantine regulations based on news from other Mediterranean ports. Tunisia was spared the severe cholera epidemics of the 1830s that struck so much of the world.

Cholera was not the only external threat feared at this time. The Ottoman government was trying to consolidate its hold on its North African territories and in 1836 asked for Tunisian military support in its imposition of direct rule in Tripoli. The aid was reluctantly sent but the bey feared Tunis would be the next Ottoman reconquest. French warships at La Goulette forestalled any possibility of this. The following year, however, French troops expanded east from Algiers occupying Constantine near the Tunisian border. The same year Ahmad Bey began his long reign (1837–55). Continuing the policies of his father and predecessor, Ahmad Bey decided to expand and modernize his army rapidly with the aid of European advisers. In 1840 he founded a military school (which still functions) at Bardo outside Tunis with Italian and French instructors. By the mid-1840s the new army was in uniforms made in factories in Tunisia. Troops were housed in European-style barracks and were equipped with imported European weapons. Conscription of Tunisian subjects replaced the importation of Ottoman or Mamluk (slave) troops. The population was heavily taxed to support the expansion and other projects undertaken by Ahmad Bey; the army was used for the first time to quell a tax revolt in the A'rad and Beja regions. Numbering 26,000, the army was a sizeable force for a population of one to one and a half million.

The beys feared the effects of epidemic diseases, which killed far more troops than swords or bullets did in the nineteenth century. Doctors were actively recruited from European states to serve in the new European-trained army. The first ones were recruited in the 1830s. An Italian, Dr Quadrini, was hired to inspect the medical facilities of the new army, and Drs Spezzafumo and Mugnaini and the British Dr Cotton were brought to serve in the artillery and infantry corps.[14] The army was to play a central and unexpected role in the spread of cholera when the disease finally invaded Tunisia.

Cholera, 1849–50, and Ahmad Bey's anxiety

In 1847 news of a serious cholera outbreak in Mecca reached Tunis. Defenses were quickly increased, but the disease soon spread by way of returning pilgrims to Egypt, Turkey, the Levant, Russia, Germany, and the rest of Europe. It was to be the beginning of a major epidemic.

On 7 January 1848 Ahmad Bey, upon instructions from the Sanitary Council, duly wrote the *amir al-liwa*'s (commanding officers) of Bizerte, Portofarina, and the other ports that suspect ships from the infected regions were not to be admitted. Nonsuspect ships were to complete a twenty-four-day quarantine, and only dry goods, thought not to carry the infection, were to be accepted. Ahmad defended his position in a general announcement:

God is kind to His people. The duty of the people is to rely on Him for preservation, to stand on the alert regarding the safety of the region, and to help the authorities in what they request and demand.... These rules are guidelines for the inspector who knows that this service is useful for the preservation of lives. Protection of all types of mankind is for us to do. From God is the preservation; it is our duty to protect ourselves.... God is the protector and the most merciful.[15]

Like Hamuda Bey, Ahmad was convinced of the value of European methods of disease prevention. This was perhaps because he thought the quarantining had worked, as cholera had in 1836 stricken many areas of Europe far more severely than Tunisia. More fundamentally, he had generally accepted the superiority of European science and technology and wanted to adopt that which made them stronger and more powerful than he was. In his letter he attempted to integrate ideas learned from the Europeans with those already held locally.[16] In standard Islamic format, he cited providence as the basis of his role as bey, therefore 'protection of all types of mankind' was his responsibility, and then he added that the quarantine authorities knew that their policies were 'useful for the preservation of lives' and should thus be obeyed. He was, however, issuing his orders on the advice of the Sanitary Council.

As elsewhere, thorough implementation of quarantines proved impossible. On 13 October 1849, for example, a Tunisian ship landed at Tabarca without permission. It had come from Bone (now Annaba) in Algeria, where the disease was suspected. After an alarmed exchange of correspondence, the boat was sent to La Goulette, where the cargo was doused with vinegar, but the crew, who had already disembarked, could have carried the disease themselves.[17]

At mid-century both Europeans and Tunisians were still uncertain as to how to protect themselves effectively. Since the mode of transmission and the causative agent of the disease were still not known, and no preventive method worked reliably, there was an unending debate over procedures. During the first pandemic, the unsanitary and poverty-stricken areas of Tunis, as elsewhere, suffered more cholera than the more affluent, cleaner quarters. This observation led many people to put their faith in the removal of noxious materials from city streets. Miasmists saw this as support for their position because fumes which caused epidemic diseases were believed to emanate from putrefying substances. Every possible means was to be applied toward the prevention of disease. From this time, the Sanitary Council included public health matters such as domestic sanitary regulations among its responsibilities.

Thomas Reade, the British consul, was, like many in his government, against the practice of quarantining. A believer in free trade, he sent Ahmad a doctor's report stating that cholera was noncontagious. Ahmad was not impressed by the argument, nor would he agree to abolish the practice of quarantine. He patiently explained to Reade:

The quarantine Regulations in our country are entrusted by us to Consuls of the Friendly Powers established in this capital. They have magnanimously agreed to establish a Quarantine on this score, as it was the case in other countries. Of course, we do not wish to have it for itself, but precautions for preserving the Public Health are of that nature which renders them both supportable and excusable, and we pray the Almighty that in His mercy He may allow us to put a stop to these measures, soon after we hear by the first arrival, that the illness has ceased.[18]

At the time of Reade's protest, Malta, which recognized British sovereignty, had been cut off from trade with Tunis after cholera appeared in Maltese cities. Since Malta was vitally dependent on trade with Tunis, this was a serious matter. The Maltese consular official who represented Reade on the Sanitary Council contacted the Foreign Office and tried to create a diplomatic incident to force the reopening of trade relations. But the bey remained adamant.

Quarantine regulations were in fact stiffened as the disease came nearer and nearer. Ships from infected regions – which by 1849 meant most European ports – had to complete forty days of quarantine elsewhere before entering the ports of Tunisia. All cargo was to be thoroughly disinfected, and letters and journals fumigated. Articles belonging to passengers were to be unloaded upon arrival and purified with vinegar.[19] The council began to meet daily rather than weekly as correspondence with the government officials became voluminous. The bey assigned his personal doctors, Lumbroso and Castelnuovo, to the council to help with deliberations and to act as his representatives. The council continued to send its recommendations to the bey or to his ministers, who then contacted the provincial governors, military officers, and port officials. The dossiers of the Sanitary Council from these years attest to the extent of shipping and the great attention given to the administration of quarantine.

Although diligent efforts were made to supervise ship quarantining, overland routes from Tripoli and Algeria were minimally controlled. When cholera broke out in eastern Algeria, a sanitary cordon was set up, but it was impossible to control all traffic in the mountainous region. The Tunisian–Algerian border was inhabited by tribes whose territories extended to both sides of the poorly defined border.[20] The tribes were in continuous communication with cholera-stricken eastern Algeria, and on 4 November 1849 the president of the Sanitary Council wrote to the bey about the illegal crossings:

I have the honor to transmit to Your Highness the information contained in a letter from the agent in Bizerte, concerning the traffic which continued to take place, by land, between Bone and Bizerte. It is my duty to observe to Your Highness how urgent it is to make a severe example against these traffikers who, in the interests of their commerce, violate the public health.[21]

Total curtailment of travel was impossible; it was too easy for people to slip across the mountainous frontier.

During the last week of November 1849 cholera broke out among the Bin Mashud tribe, which lived on both sides of the Tunisian–Algerian border,[22] and spread to the Awlad Nafal in Raqaba, near Beja, a major city in the western region. The government ordered a cordon around the infected tribespeople. This cordon was policed by individuals from the tribe itself;[23] it is unlikely that those who saw no clear reason for such

46

a cordon would have been diligent in its enforcement. Whether or not the cordon was enforced, the disease soon spread to other regions. Ahmad Bey sent an Italian doctor to investigate reports of cholera and dispatched troops to prevent more people from entering his territories from Algeria. On 23 November 1849 the disease was reported among the Janduba tribe near Suq al-Khamis, where eighteen persons died within a few days. The doctor wrote to Lumbroso in Tunis to say that while cholera did exist, he had been unable to reach the infected regions because of heavy rains. The disease had spread during six days of cold, frost, hail, and violent rains.[24]

The bey had taken these steps without consulting the Sanitary Council. On 2 December the council sent the bey a resentful reproach:

The Council of Health has learned by the public voice the sad news of the appearance of cholera in a region of the interior. In regretting that Your Highness had not given official knowledge to news that so much interests the public health, we urge you to send a commission of competent and experienced doctors to the place, and to carefully examine the sickness and to take precautions and remedies which could immediately extinguish the foyer and prevent its expansion to the rest of the Regency.[25]

The bey was deluged with complaints from the Sanitary Council and reports from the local authorities informing him of the disease in their regions. More troops were sent to the stricken regions. Two people died in Tunis of suspicious symptoms, causing great alarm. One was a Maltese who had arrived from Beja two days earlier. He was diagnosed as having succumbed to the effects of a 'long and arduous journey, indigestible food, and a considerable amount of spirits'. The other victim was a man from the Jewish community in Tunis who was taken to the hospital of the Sisters of Saint Joseph, where his fatal illness was diagnosed as 'natural intestinal poisoning'. The population was reassured and calmed for the moment.[26]

In anticipation of the epidemic reaching Tunis, the bey had three barracks adapted for use as temporary hospitals,[27] one for Muslims, one for Jews, and the third for Catholics. The shaykh al-madina was also to see to the enforcement of the measures suggested by the Sanitary Council for cleaning the city streets. The council also requested that the bey rescind the tax on meat, as protein was considered the best fortification in time of illness, but this was not carried out.[28]

On 3 December Ahmad sent another doctor, Mancel, to Beja, as there was news that the disease was spreading rapidly. He reported that it was impossible to judge the extent of the disease because neither the *kahiya* (deputy officer) nor the European doctor were there and the shaykhs gave him no information.[29] But he said that the disease did seem to be spreading: 'One can count four or five deaths and at least forty sick, judging from the great number of unhappy, frightened people who come from everywhere to look for me.' After several days Mancel collected sufficient information to convince the Sanitary Council that an epidemic existed, and cholera was officially declared in the region.

After this declaration Ahmad announced measures for the protection of Tunis, which was to be cordoned off from the infected areas. He again ordered the shaykhs of the city to supervise the street cleaning, for which money was collected. While these preparations were under way, the amir al-liwa' of the cavalry was dispatched with troops to form a cordon along the left bank of the Majerda River, which cut Tunis off from the west and north. The bey sent strict orders to the local authorities of rural towns to segregate the Bedouin encampments from the towns.[30]

In Tunis prices immediately rose as a result of the cordon. The Sanitary Council complained to the bey that he had violated his agreement by allowing the rise in prices; but there was little the bey could do to avoid a scarcity of foodstuffs while the cordon was in effect.[31] The council went on to suggest again that the tax on meat be dropped and also encouraged the bey to find other means of bringing in foodstuffs. It informed the bey that the tax cut would 'have a healthy moral effect upon a population which would be plunged into a profound discouragement by its isolation from the Chief of State, if the effects of the promises [to control prices] were not immediately felt'.[32]

The council referred to the fact that the bey had isolated himself upon the first news of the epidemic. This was on the advice of his personal physician, Abraham Lumbroso, a member of a prominent Livornese–Jewish family of Tunis. Lumbroso was to play a central role in the cholera epidemic and was in an excellent position to observe matters of public health in Tunisia. His books about the epidemic and general conditions in Tunisia are eloquent and perceptive and are invaluable sources of information. His *Cenni storico-scientifici sul cholera-morbus asiatico che invase la reggenza di Tunis nel 1849–1850* and *Lettres médico-statistiques sur la régence de Tunis* are primary sources for this study.[33]

Terrorized by the spreading epidemic, on 5 December Ahmad Bey moved to a residence in the gardens of his minister, Mustafa Khaznadar, in Carthage. He took along his personal retinue and a guard of soldiers to camp in tents around the residence. He then ordered the minister of war to move to neighboring al-Kram so that he could meet with the bey every day.[34]

With cholera spreading through the western regions, few expected

Tunis to be spared, despite its cordon of troops. On 17 December 1849 a traveling merchant fell ill and died in the *hara* (Jewish quarter) two days later. The same night, his mother-in-law, who had been called in to assist, also fell ill. Then the sickness jumped to another house. Soon the disease was spreading through the quarter. Lumbroso described the early stages of the outbreak:

[The disease] spread to nearby houses, all inhabited by Jews, as if that germ had some sort of knowledge and avoided all other sects except the Jews. We eventually had a mortality of about fifty persons out of about 150–200 stricken every day. If fear had not imposed itself on this stricken nation, forcing them to emigrate abroad or to other regions of the Regency, perhaps the number of victims might have been much higher.[35]

Bin Diyaf also noted that the initial appearance of the disease was in the hara: 'It happened that when the disease descended upon the capital, it first befell among poor Jews, and the catastrophe was very serious. Man fled his brother, his mother and father, his wife and his sons....'[36]

The occurrence of the disease in the hara was difficult for the doctors to explain. If there was an epidemic of cholera, why was it limited to the Jewish population? One of the doctors who opposed the diagnosis of cholera called on the shaykh al-madina, who took him to visit three sick persons in the hara. After seeing them, he diagnosed gastroenteric disturbance and observed that the Jews had just fasted for three days and had then eaten an excess of such foods as beets and carrots. The doctor had been in Tunisia during the 1836 outbreak of cholera and also during a typhus epidemic and noted that neither epidemic had discriminated among Muslims, Jews, and Christians. Furthermore, he reasoned, in the virulent outbreak of cholera in the Beja region, many Muslims were perishing. In Beja itself, there had already been fifteen hundred deaths, and in the Zawiya of al-Madyani, there had been a hundred and fifty victims among the four hundred who lived there. In ten days in Le Kef, twelve hundred had died. 'Is it possible,' he asked, 'for this disease, in such a city as Tunis, populated as it is by different ethnic groups, to stay a whole month with the Jews who are amalgamated with and surrounded by the others?'[37]

In the light of current knowledge concerning the mode of transmission of cholera, it is not difficult to understand why the disease spread as it did. Cholera spreads most frequently by means of contaminated water supplies, and Tunis was organized into quarters which were relatively separate from each other. The hara was an impoverished, unsanitary, overcrowded section of the city and when the disease first broke out among its residents, it could have easily contaminated the public water supply and thus spread rapidly throughout the quarter. The traveling merchant may have contracted the disease outside the quarter and then communicated it by direct or indirect contact to the rest of the inhabitants. The custom of gathering in a room of the deceased probably aided transmission of the disease via the food and water of the household.

The peculiar spread of the disease by ethnic group was noted by the residents of the city, who made it the basis of a tale about the origins of the disease. The tale also indicates an awareness of the route by which cholera entered Tunisia:

The cholera, after having passed from France to Algeria, went from this last country to Tunis. While still on the road, he arrived at Carthage and met the marabout of Sidi bu Said. Sensing the imminent danger to the Muslims of Tunis, who were under his protection, the saint awoke from his long sleep and said,

'Where are you going, Oh bold one?'

'To Tunis.'

'What for?'

'For what I do everywhere! I need victims!'

'Well then, take them from the Jews, take them from the Christians too. I hold neither the one nor the other dear. As for the Muslims, they are mine. I cannot bear that you touch them.'

This was agreed. The cholera pursued his journey. He was soon before the chapel of Saint Louis, the French saint. He was no less jealous of the health of his co-religionists. He also rose from his tomb and asked the cholera, 'Oh unhappy one, where are you going?'

'You know where! To Tunis!'

The saint replied, 'I am the protector of the Christians of Tunis. You must respect them. You must not touch them.'

This was agreed. The cholera again took up his route, which led directly to Tunis leaving La Goulette [the predominantly Jewish suburb] to the left. If he had only encountered another saint who was the protector of the Jewish nation, he might not have entered the city at all.[38]

The disease entered Tunis, and the barracks previously designated as hospitals were opened on 27 December to aid the stricken quarter. Doctors from the *nizam jadid* (the new European-style Tunisian army) were assigned to the hospitals, and daily statistics were collected. Lumbroso prepared medical instructions for the people of Tunis as well as for the rural nomadic tribes. Copies were printed in Italian and Arabic and distributed in the churches and mosques. The instructions were, as Lumbroso claimed, adapted to 'national custom' and divided into three categories: personal hygiene, cleanliness of homes, and diet.[39]

During the first weeks of January 1850 a few cases of cholera occurred among the Muslims. *Mawlid al-nabiy*, the Prophet's birthday, fell that year on 27 January, and there was hesitation as to whether the mawlid celebration should be held in the bey's absence and with the disease distressing people. But Ahmad wrote from his palace in Carthage, ordering that the congregation and other rituals be held as usual. For this purpose, he ordered oil to be sent to the minarets. The meeting was held, cannons fired, and two verses from the Quran read 'to comfort the people in time of difficulty'.[40]

Following the holiday ceremonies, the epidemic spread rapidly in the Muslim quarters, suggesting that the crowds in close contact hastened transmission of the disease. Muhammad Sharif, one of the more respected notables of the city, died on 6 February, followed by several members of his family and others who had visited him.[41] Soon the disease was raging throughout the city.

The appearance of the new disease caused a reaction by ordinary people against European and Muslim elites. As the symptoms of cholera strongly resemble those of poisoning, people everywhere suspected foul play rather than epidemic disease. Mancel, who had been sent to Beja, was accused of this:

There were still true sons of Satan who belonged to high society who tried to spread the seeds of revolt. These people said that the French doctor [Mancel] was wrong [in his diagnosis of cholera]. His defects were that he was very poor and had sold himself to the government which for political reasons wanted to create alarm among its people. Others suspected that various *qa'id*s [governors] were promulgating these alarms to exempt themselves from taxes due, and their French doctor was making himself their accomplice. Still others said that all doctors were bought and were spreading poisons for the total destruction of human beings wherever possible.[42]

But such suspicions and accusations could not stop the course of the disease. Popular agitation against medical personnel persisted, to the anger of Lumbroso:

This gave rise to incidents in which the doctors were threatened or even manhandled, and very idiotic satires were directed at them. So bad were these defamatory rumors that it became the cause of the greater spread and longer duration of the epidemic since when it appeared in the capital the poor and ignorant believed these rumors and did not seek medical assistance which they feared. It reached such a point that we heard curses hurled at those who had taken medicines prescribed by the doctors.[43]

Popular opinion was in general suspicious of European doctors and, by extension, of their medicine. In one incident, which was reported in a French newspaper, Dr Mancel was thought to have brought the disease to Bizerte. On 12 March 1850 seven of the eight he had treated died. Mancel was accused of having caused their sickness by his breath and his glance. A light fog which had been noticed over some stagnant water in the area where the deaths occurred was also attributed to him. A riot subsequently broke out and the doctor fled the town.[44]

Ahmad's self-isolation, which he carried to the extreme and which was instigated on Lumbroso's advice, was also publicly criticized. After his long absence, rumors circulated that the bey had secretly left the kingdom. There were threats of urban disturbances. In order to allay the rumors, Ahmad began to go out in front of the palace in which he had isolated himself, and 'even got near the guard's tents so the people could see him'. Bin Diyaf himself complained about Ahmad's extreme measures. Letters were brought to the head guard's tent, where they were opened and copied by a scribe. The copy was flamed and then taken to the bey; the original was burned. All business with the outside was conducted by letter. Bin Diyaf, the bey's secretary, found the burden tedious even with the assistance of another scribe.[45]

One day Bin Diyaf had a conversation with the bey during which he reproached him for his fear of the epidemic. Ahmad replied:

Fear is disgraceful when you can see the opponent and it can see you and you can touch it and it can touch you. When it is the power of God Almighty, if fear is not appropriate, neither is it shameful. Perhaps courage in such matters is lack of respect before God as we would not be placing ourselves in his Hands.... If divine decree and fate arrive and I die with this disease, I fear I would say 'if only I had observed the quarantine, this would not have happened', because of my belief that everything comes from God.[46]

Ahmad thus combined his natural desire for self-preservation and his belief in medical advice from his European doctor with a defense based on divine providence. He then cited a letter the noted *'alim* (religious scholar) Shaykh Muhammad Bayram had composed for his uncle on the permissibility of protection from such an epidemic, as further evidence of the validity of his position (see p. 31).

A group of Ahmad's ministers criticized him for his actions, saying, 'Precaution by means of "quarantine" was not found in the religion of Islam but was an invention of Christendom, and we know better than the Christians the ways of the disease'. But Ahmad would not listen to them and only increased his vigilance.[47]

A debate that followed recalls opinions held by Muslims since the earliest days of Islam. Mustafa Khaznadar, the Mamluk treasurer, citing various hadiths, asserted that those who died of cholera were martyrs. He was implying that extensive public medical assistance and the quarantine were not necessary. It may be assumed that Khaznadar resented both the interereference with lucrative commercial ventures and the expenditure of state funds for the relief effort because this curtailed his own embezzlement of state funds. Bin Diyaf took the opposite position, that protection from epidemic disease was legal, and stated that there was no legal text that disproved it. The two then sought the opinion of certain 'ulama'. Tayib al-Riyahi, the learned son and expected successor of the famous reformer Ibrahim al-Riyahi, the imam of the Great Mosque, gave his opinion that 'victims of cholera were martyrs as they were *mabtun* or suffering from internal wounds, as in the hadith of [the Maliki law book] the *Muwatta*''. Khaznadar and Bin Diyaf then went to the mufti, Muhammad b. Salama, who argued that the victims of cholera were not martyrs. Bin Diyaf ended his discussion with the cryptic observation that in any case both of the 'alims died of cholera.[48]

The bey's fears increased when cases of the disease were announced in Carthage; he decided to move to Muhammadiya, which had until then been free of cholera. He had considered going to Djerba, but his ministers convinced him that the island was too remote. On 20 February the entire retinue moved to Muhammadiya, where Ahmad's palace was being constructed.[49]

A week after his departure, the disease began to abate in Tunis and the temporary hospitals were closed down. Most people evidently preferred to be cared for at home. From 27 December 1849 to 20 February 1850 the hospitals had served only 169 people.[50] According to the statistics brought to Lumbroso by the shaykhs of the city and the doctors working in the hospitals, about 1,900 of the 15,000 Jews of the capital had perished of 3,700 cases, as had about 900 of the 85,000 or 100,000 Muslims of 2,400 cases.[51] There had also been a high mortality in the interior, where the disease still existed.

The Sanitary Council, however, felt that the worst was over and asked the bey to authorize the establishment of a permanent hospital in the center of town. The hospital would provide services in addition to those of the maristan, which was very small and functioned mainly as a hospice for the mentally ill and a place for the preparation of corpses for burial. The council suggested that the hospital be placed in communication with one located in the European quarter, where the Sisters of Charity exercised their very useful ministrations.[52]

Ahmad evidently planned to expand the temporary hospitals and establish a permanent hospital and even a medical school. He was aware of similar developments in Egypt under his contemporary, Muhammad 'Ali. Shortly after the cholera epidemic, Clot Bey, Muhammad 'Ali's chief doctor, hearing of Ahmad's interest, sent Ahmad a shipment of medical books he had had translated into Arabic and included a letter describing his achievements in the field of medicine in Egypt.[53] The cholera epidemic thus contributed to the implantation of European medicine, though the hospital and medical school remained only a plan during Ahmad's reign.

The disease, thought to be on the wane at the end of February 1850, suddenly reappeared in Tunis during the last days of March. But it was not serious enough to alarm the authorities, and the sanitary cordons that had been discontinued were not reinstated. Trade and travel were carried on freely, and at the end of March a battalion of troops which had been confined to Tunis were allowed to disperse. Most of the troops lived in the Sahel, and a few days after their return home, the disease was rampant in the cities and towns of that region. The tribes living around Kairouan were severely stricken. By mid-June Mahdiya, with 6,000 inhabitants, lost about 300 of them to cholera, and many more were sick. Local authorities in Gabes estimated about 2,000 had perished in a few days, and the Djerid region was reported to have lost about 8,000 persons.[54]

Cholera had broken out among the 800 troops guarding Ahmad's refuge in Muhammadiya. In panic, Ahmad departed for Portofarina, where the disease had not yet appeared. He had no sooner arrived than the disease was found among the crew of the *Minos*,[55] the ship that had taken him to Portofarina. Nevertheless, the bey stayed there, as the disease had flared up again in Tunis and he no longer had anywhere to go.[56]

The second outbreak of cholera in Tunis, which occurred during the spring and summer of 1850, was even more virulent than the first. All quarters of the city were immediately affected, and mortality rates were higher as well. The European doctors continued to debate the manner of the spread of the disease. Some, including Lumbroso, were convinced contagionists, but when the disease was found in the interior but not in Tunis during the months of February and March, Lumbroso was forced to explain this as a result of unknown cosmo-tellurgical reasons. He suggested that miasmas were perhaps to blame, because more people died in the plains and swampy areas than in the mountains.[57] Doctors were baffled when cholera reappeared in Tunis, having disappeared for several weeks.

The temporary hospitals reopened on 15 June and remained open until 4 August 1850. The disease attacked all communities with equal fervor during this second stage. The relief committees were reorganized. Lumbroso listed the following charities provided by the bey during the epidemic:[58]

200	qafiz of grain
300	tins of oil
60	suits of clothing for individuals of formerly well-off families
60	suits of clothing for needy artisans
60	suits of work clothes for the poor
180	*safsaris* [shawls] for needy women
12,000	piasters plus the necessary materials for fumigation. The large, well-equipped hospital directed by a commission of naval doctors and other doctors of experience.

The meager donations helped but a few hundred persons in the capital city. The hospitals served only a small part of the population of Tunis, and no similar hospitals were set up outside the capital. According to Lumbroso's statistics, only 455 people were admitted to the hospitals during the two stages of the epidemic; 266 of them died.[59] This number represents a mortality rate of 60 percent, higher than the mortality rate of those not served by the hospitals. It is likely that only those suffering from the last stages of the illness were willing to be taken there.

Despite all the medical efforts, cholera was still rampant toward the end of June 1850. Ahmad Bey decided to take further steps to halt the epidemic and ordered the Hanafi *qadi* (judge), Muhammad b. Husayn Bayram, to arrange an invocation. He ordered forty *sharif*s (descendants of the Prophet) who were named Muhammad to convene daily at the Great Mosque from morning until noon to read the Quranic Sura 'Ya Sin' forty times and to invoke God with a special du'a' which the qadi prepared from selected holy works. The bey gave the signal for the beginning of the invocation, and it proceeded as ordered.[60] An example of one of the invocations used during the 1850 epidemic, composed by Mahmud Qabadu, the noted scholar, poet, and reformer, reads as follows:

> . . . .
> You brought us into your confines
> . . . .
> You are the merciful and our mercy.
> You are compassionate when angry with your creatures.
> Your power has superiority over the feverish.
> You who possess all possession.
> We have no means or power save through your all powerful will.
> You who created medicine; it is shameful for our hearts and bodies to complain about our misery. . . .[61]

Just after the invocation was made at the Great Mosque, the disease abated and soon disappeared. The apparent effectiveness of this measure was such that Mustafa Khaznadar announced that the men who participated in the invocation no longer needed proof of their holy descent.[62] The epidemic was officially declared over by the Sanitary Council the first week of August. Patents of ships leaving the ports of Tunisia were acordingly marked 'clean' and normal trade and travel resumed. The religious measure must have seemed to many responsible for the final disappearance of the disease.[63] Or could Muslim or European practitioners take credit? Had their medicine proven effective?

To his surprise Lumbroso observed that indigenous empirics were as successful as European doctors in treating cholera.[64] Most, he found, preferred external treatment and administration of bland and oily mixtures, potions of aromatic herbs, olive oil, and honey, and doses of vinegar and garlic.[65] In Algeria Bertherand observed that 'the *tabibs* [doctors] used *chenedegoura* [ground ivy], olive oil, and water drunk in large quantities. They covered the abdomen with large stones or heated earthen dishes. They massaged the feet and parts of the body seized with cramps, always with success.' Dr Loir-Montgazon wrote to Bertherand informing him of his experience in the Tunisian Sahara during the limited outbreak of 1836. 'The tabibs began by rapidly touching red hot iron needles to the stomach; then they covered the patient in warm wool covers, and finally made him drink a hot infusion of flowers of *vipérine bâtarde* [borage] found in abundance in the countryside.... I have to state that the scarifications on the stomach have produced before me such happy results that I have often continued the usage. The application of this powerful derivative stops the vomiting almost instantly and alleviates in a sensible manner the stomach pains.'[66]

Like European treatments, Muslim medical treatments were essentially symptomatic. But Muslims adapted older medical concepts to the new disease while European researchers were trying to discover the causative agent by means of experimental methodologies. In one Muslim version of the etiology of cholera, the various manifestations of the disease were neatly but unproductively accounted for:

Five janun were responsible for cholera. The first, Aya'il, had a list with the names of those condemned to death. Those who died barely stricken had been hit by the arrows of the second jinn, Ya'il. Those who died on the first day after sudden illness were hit in the heart by arrows of the third jinn, Haiha'il. If an abscess appeared on the skin of the victim, it was the result of wounds from arrows of the fourth jinn, Griha'il. The fifth jinn, Shaykha'il, was armed with clubs and stones and killed by striking the victim in the heart, stomach or head, causing accumulation of blood in the mouth, altered reason, prolonged suffering, loss of speech, and slow death. Those who were stricken and recovered did not have their names on Aya'il's list; their time had not come. Regions not stricken were spared because the jinn did not receive orders to strike.[67]

Correct understanding of the cause of cholera was not of course necessary for treatment. Muslim doctors relied primarily on scarification and potions of herbs and olive oil. Like their European counterparts, they could only prescribe their remedies and hope for the best.

The cholera-stricken were correct in their mistrust of European doctors for the treatments they favored were at best next to useless and at worst deadly. Lumbroso listed various treatments used by European doctors during the epidemic. Maschero, a Spanish doctor who had been assigned to a temporary hospital, bled his patients at the first symptoms, and if they worsened he opted for emetics. To induce vomiting, he used olive oil and in a few cases prescribed touching the epigastric region with a hot iron, treatments probably learned from the Muslim doctors.

Ferrini, an Italian doctor, considered the use of caloric (a substance then thought to contain the properties of heat) indispensable. It was to be placed in a bladder which was then put on the patient's stomach; the bladder was used to keep the caloric from running over the extremities of the body. For a person predisposed to cholera, that is, one with a sanguine temperament (a concept derived from Greek medical theory) or with habitual dysentery, Ferrini prescribed bloodletting as a necessary precaution. He too used emetics when symptoms called for it to 'replace diarrhea with violent vomiting'. If the patient was in the last stages of cold, he fed him oil of camomile or other mild substances. If the patient was threatened with suffocation, he thought bloodletting mandatory! Lumbroso himself favored applying mustard plaster to the extremities with friction, using a woolen cloth soaked with hot water and acetic acid. Dr Cotton preferred external treatments, purgatives, vomitives, narcotics, and emetics. He did not like using opium for fear of congestion and brain and lung inflammation. During the period of cold, he placed his patients in a very hot bath and covered them with mustard plaster. He felt that bleeding was at that time 'unpleasant and dangerous'. He also used quinine (derived from cinchona root, a Peruvian folk remedy effective against malaria) in heavy doses.[68]

One can only pity the cholera victim of those decades. Europeans and Muslims alike imagined that bleeding removed excess blood and allowed the heart more easily to pump the remaining blood. But bleeding was the worst treatment imaginable for the disease that caused death by dehydration from vomiting and diarrhea. British doctors used the deadly practice in India during the first outbreaks of cholera of the nineteenth century. According to a frequently cited report, bleeding was considered the most successful treatment during the first cholera pandemic (1829–34). The purgatives, emetics, and vomitives likewise served only to hasten the death of the patient by increasing dehydration. It was only toward the end of the nineteenth century and after repeated experience with the poor results of these treatments that less harsh methods came into vogue.[69]

Sometimes, European and Muslim medical theories and practices were synthesized. European medical ideas came directly to Tunisia not only from Europeans who held positions of authority, but also through the existing Ottoman power structure centered in Istanbul. Tunisia was formally part of the Ottoman Empire and Istanbul was a prominent intellectual and political center. This gave credence to a treatise on cholera written in 1831 by Mustafa Behçet, the *bash hakim* (chief physician) of Istanbul.[70] Behçet was trained in the Muslim medical college of Istanbul, but he had also learned several European languages and was interested in and familiar with recent European medical ideas. His treatise was based on an Austrian manual on cholera but was adapted for use in Ottoman regions and was written in the classical tradition of Islamic medicine.[71]

Behçet's treatise contained a brief history of cholera, stating that the disease had begun in India and had traveled from country to country. Behçet ascribed the symptoms to the burning of the bile and said that since cholera was not described in the medical books of the ancient doctors, it was incumbent upon him to write the treatise. After an accurate description of the symptoms of the disease, he recommended bleeding, following standard European treatment. A convinced contagionist, Behçet said the disease could be transmitted from person to person like plague. He suggested holding vinegar, garlic, or ammonia to one's face as protection from the contagion. For this purpose, he also recommended burning tar, incense, gum arabic, pine leaves, and other aromatic plants found in the Mediterranean and traditionally used in Muslim medical practice to purify the air.

The treatise was translated from Turkish into Arabic in Tunis and seems to have enjoyed wide circulation, judging by the number of copies preserved in the national library of Tunis and elsewhere. It was copied as a separate work or kept with other manuscripts dealing with magical remedies and du'a's especially for use against epidemics. Such books were evidently kept on hand for reference when needed.

None of the European accounts of the cholera epidemics in Tunisia mention the existence of this Arabic- and Turkish-language treatise on cholera. In all probability, however, it served as an important source of current European medical knowledge to a Muslim readership. A skillful combination of Muslim medical practice and nineteenth-century European knowledge, Behçet's treatise might be considered another means of borrowing European knowledge, in this case through Istanbul and Ottoman medical authority rather than through direct European contact.

Mortality rates for those treated by European and Muslim practitioners do not appear to have differed significantly. General care and comfort were the only effective aids most doctors were able to provide before the medical innovations of the twentieth century. Before treatments with antibiotic medicines and intravenous feeding were discovered, mortality from cholera was generally about 40 to 60 percent.

Cholera, 1856, and an anti-European bey

Cholera returned again in epidemic form in 1856, during the reign of Ahmad's cousin and successor, Muhammad Bey (1855–9). Muhammad Bey disliked Western-style reforms and did everything he could to restore the old order. He reduced taxes to legal Islamic levels, disbanded the Westernized army, and even moved French furniture from his palace.

Muhammad Bey's actions at the outbreak of cholera were a sharp contrast to those of his predecessor. At the beginning the quarantine service organized by the Sanitary Council functioned as it had during the earlier cholera threats. News of a threat first reached Tunis in July 1856, when the kahiya of the island of Djerba wrote to Isma'il Sahib al-Taba' to inform him that cholera had broken out in Tripoli and that the shaykhs or authorities of the island had had a meeting in its capital, Humt Suq, had decided to defend themselves against people coming from infected regions, and had therefore placed guards on the beaches. A few months earlier the kahiya had written to say that a ship loaded with pilgrims was coming from the east and that the authorities, greatly alarmed, had increased their guard. A boat with twelve armed guards was sent out to patrol the waters to prevent illegal landings. One night a caravan of Bedouins waded over a shallow place in the water called 'road of camels' but were caught just as they were reching the island. A skirmish resulted and seven men and eight camels were caught. The kahiya heard that some of those who had escaped were lost at sea and the rest had reached the mainland. Those who were captured were put in quarantine and later transferred to jail. The Djerban authorities in the 1850s clearly had no doubt as to the disease's contagiousness nor about the necessity of maintaining the quarantine.[72]

But Muhammad Bey did. When, despite all precautions, the disease did invade and spread north to Tunis, Muhammad Bey refused to implement any of the measures recommended by the Sanitary Council. He also refused to quarantine himself or his children and continued to mingle with the public. His insistence on visiting the sick in his palace without fear of contagion greatly encouraged people. Bin Diyaf counted this among his good deeds in a eulogy following his death in 1860. Bin Diyaf further observed that the 1856 cholera epidemic was less severe and of shorter duration than the earlier epidemic, when Ahmad Bey had taken such energetic precautions.[73]

Muhammad Bey authorized none of the preventive measures nor treatment centers initiated during the 1849–50 epidemic. Since the epidemic occurred in August, most of the European doctors were out of the country. Medical treatments practiced in Tunisia had not evolved significantly in the five years following the previous epidemic and need not be repeated here. They were no less and no more effective; the disease played itself out and vanished for a decade.

Social and economic consequences of cholera, 1830–58

William McNeill, in *Plagues and Peoples*, has suggested that 'the unfamiliar, dreadful, and sudden nature of cholera deaths created among the population of Egypt and other affected Moslem lands almost the same alarm that prevailed in Europe. Neither Moslem medical nor religious traditions were able to cope. The popular fright cholera aroused helped to discredit traditional leadership and authority within the Moslem world, and opened the way for reception of European medicine.'[74] Did cholera in Tunisia have this effect? Certainly the alarm was real, but it does not appear that European medical (or religious) traditions were better able to cope at this time than their Muslim counterparts. Cholera was a new disease to Muslim doctors, but they used standard symptomatic treatments for dysentery and fever. There is no evidence that traditional authorities were discredited by their failure to combat cholera in Tunisia. Moreover, the effectiveness of the forty sharifs named Muhammad in vitiating the epidemic should have reinforced confidence in received religious traditions. If it was not popular observance of the superiority of European medical ability in coping with epidemics that opened the way for the reception of European medicine, what was it?

European medicine had been sought by the beys since at least the eighteenth century. European science in general had proven itself in many areas and the superior effectiveness of European medicine against all ailments, including epidemic diseases, was a rational deduction. And European medicine was associated with new sources of political power which the beys hoped to rival. Thus, the adoption of European medicine, stimulated by the crises presented by the epidemics and by new political and social perceptions, began at elite levels in the face of popular disapproval and distrust.

The Westernizing beys were, in fact, condemned by the populace for their reliance on European guidance, for their expensive reform programs, for their increased taxes, and for their association with nontraditional authorities to the detriment of local interests, sympathies, and sensibilities. With the exception of the very small Europeanized elite, the majority of the population remained apart from the European doctors and continued to follow the medical beliefs of their ancestors. This was in part the result of their conviction that their ways were satisfactory for themselves and superior to those of Europeans, and in part a reaction to the disadvantageous ways being forced upon them. Most, of course, had no direct personal contact with the handful of European doctors then in Tunisia but saw no clear gain from the European presence.

The general suspicion with which the Europeans were regarded was manifested in the belief that they could cause disease or had been bought by the ruler and therefore gave biased diagnoses. During the cholera epidemic of 1849–50 European doctors had been accused of causing the disease with their glance or breath, or starting rumors to cause panic. Muslims who had previously sought European medical advice refused to consult European doctors altogether. Occasionally European doctors were roughed up by the crowds. The few Muslims who persisted in consulting European doctors were occasionally included in the condemnation. Sometimes there were confrontations between European and indigenous doctors. The persistence of traditional beliefs concerning the origin of epidemic disease infuriated Dr Lumbroso:

One finds in our time, some poor souls who believe in all good faith that all pestilential epidemic disease is born of the letting loose of a diabolical army, whose soldiers ravage the whole country – sometimes one, sometimes another.... Some say they have clearly seen them, others have only heard their voices, finally one has been followed by them in a dream.[75]

Lumbroso had only scorn for the Sufi practitioners who were called in to exorcise the jinn, calling them 'charlatans and cheats who wish to profit from deceit'.[76]

The meeting of the two systems of medical perception when it occurred among ordinary people resulted in mutual disregard. To Lumbroso's intense annoyance, he and his colleagues were often asked to cede to a local Muslim doctor their place at the bedside of the seriously ill.[77] Ahmad Bey, however, made his own preference clear. Lumbroso had, by the 1840s, become a member of the bey's most trusted inner circle. The government of France also courted his favor, awarding him in 1846 the Cross of the Legion of Honor and nominating him to the Order of Saint Lazare. In 1856 he was to be appointed consul of San Marino, an ideal appointment for the Italian city-state since he had direct access to the bey. Lumbroso represented its commercial community at court and as one of the bey's closest advisers was able actively to promote merchants' interests. The dual position of this doctor reflects not only Ahmad's faith in European medicine but also the emerging importance of Italians in Tunisian affairs.[78]

Moreover, the Sanitary Council, composed of consuls acting in advisory capacity to the beys, had itself become a political force. The members of the council fought over medical and economic issues with the lines of conflict reflecting not only medical but also political rationales. The council was an active organization that met frequently, kept voluminous records, and eventually subsumed what had been a central responsibility of the ruler. The fact that the members were representatives of foreign commercial and political interests rather than medical authorities from the local government indicates a marked shift in official priorities.

During the last years of his reign, however, Ahmad Bey suspected that his Europeanization policies had become unmanageable. According to Bin Diyaf, he frequently asked who was running his country, he or the European consuls.[79] In the early 1850s he repeatedly tried to overrule the decisions of the Sanitary Council. Sometimes disputes arose over the quarantining of ships; letters between ships' captains, their consuls, and Ahmad are preserved in the government archives of Tunis. Ahmad usually insisted on more stringent quarantines than the Sanitary Council felt were necessary. The correspondence even extended to minute details: Ahmad insisted that letters be opened and disinfected with perfume of chloride, while the council, probably in an effort to protect the secrecy of official correspondence, insisted that the perfuming be done through an incision in the envelope.[80] The essence of such arguments was not only personal safety but also the question of power, and Ahmad took every opportunity to assert his authority over those he thought were challenging his supremacy.

The Sanitary Council repeatedly accused Ahmad of enacting contradictory and inconsistent measures that had caused trouble with governments 'friendly to the Bey'. They demanded that the original guidelines be followed and that the Sanitary Council be accorded complete jurisdiction in the administration of the quarantine.[81] In 1855, the last year of Ahmad's reign, the council complained to the bey that although they had been meeting for twenty years and had taken care to employ 'all measures outside the Regency, he, the bey, kept overruling their authority'.[82]

It cannot be said that the inability of Muslim medical and religious traditions to cope with cholera discredited them with the public. On the contrary, it was Ahmad Bey and other members of the elite who, despite misgivings, were beginning to demonstrate new faith in European science and in European doctors. If anything, it was their reliance on European advice and support that tended to discredit them in public opinion. This was to change as Europeans became the dominant political force.

The cholera epidemic of 1849–50 had come at a time of serious economic difficulty. The bey's military reforms and construction projects undertaken to redress the balance of power were expensive. The balance of trade was severely upset by imposed commercial agreements. Though cholera did not cause mortality comparable to the earlier plague epidemics – at most a tenth of the population perished – it was a major disaster. Like the 1818–20 plague epidemic, cholera was associated by contemporaries with a depression in agriculture. Poor harvests and famine followed on the heels of the epidemic. According to Bin Diyaf, agriculture almost ceased and 'even the wild animals' were dying. In addition, military troops had been badly hit by the epidemic and in 1850, when the bey ordered a new conscription for additional recruits, the population was sorely tested. They were, in Bin Diyaf's words, 'still reeling from the crisis'.[83]

The situation worsened in 1852 when Bin 'Ayad, the minister of finance, fled to Paris with state funds to which he had access. This nearly bankrupted the already weak treasury. Efforts to retrieve the funds proved unsuccessful. Because of lack of funds, the army was in part disbanded, and one after another of the military factories closed down. Tunisian participation in the Crimean War of 1854–5 was a further drain on the budget; Ahmad Bey had to sell most of his jewels to finance the venture. Some 4,000 of the nearly 10,000 troops sent perished from epidemic diseases in the camps.[84]

Like earlier epidemics, however, the 1849–50 cholera outbreak cannot be called a direct cause of economic reversals. The 1849–50 epidemic was part of a pandemic that struck most regions of Europe, Asia, and America and recovery was rapid in most of those regions. Tunisia was, at the time, in the midst of a depression aggravated by the commercial domination of the European merchants and consuls, and by the expensive military programs initiated in response by the bey. The early 1850s were difficult years, and the epidemic only added to the existing hardship.

The epidemic of 1856 was of shorter duration than the previous one but was severe in Tunis, Beja, and parts of the Sahel. But it was followed by a spell of prosperity. Muhammad Bey was able to lighten taxes by reducing the size of the army and just after the epidemic, announced a regularization of tax laws so that the *fallahin* (peasants) knew in advance exactly how much they were to pay. They result was rapid expansion of agriculture in 1857–8, aided by favorable weather. This brought a quick, though temporary, reversal in Tunisia's fortunes.[85]

Despite the attitude of Muhammad Bey, the reforms in public health and medicine were there to stay. The experience with cholera of 1849–50 had led to new European and Muslim political efforts in the field of medicine: formation of the Sanitary Council, extension of the quarantine network, the *ad hoc* hospitals directed by European military doctors, the as yet unrealized plans for a medical school, and the scientific studies of epidemics by Lumbroso and others.

Muhammad Bey's actions in refusing to follow European-style precautions in the face of cholera epidemic may have won him a measure of public approval, but he was unable to avoid all innovations. In 1858 Muhammad Bey authorized the creation of a Municipal Council, on the recommendation of the Sanitary Council, which was responsible for the upkeep of public buildings, maintenance of roads, and supervision of traffic.[86] The first president of the council was Husayn Sharif, who served from 1858 to 1865. He was succeeded by Muhammad Qara, al-'Arbi Zarruq, and Hassuna Dali, who resigned in 1882 when the French administration assumed direct control. Muhammad Bey had tried to resist but, in the end, as will be seen in Chapter 3, he instituted more substantial Europeanizing reforms than had Ahmad Bey. And Muhammad Bey himself asked the French consul to send him a doctor during his last illness.[87]

One might have observed that European medical procedures contributed little to the eradication of cholera, but despite uncertainty and apprehension the Muslim elite had decided they were superior to indigenous methods. This reflected the increasingly dominant role Europeans were playing in Tunisian affairs. European doctors were in subsequent years to replace indigenous ones in all official capacities. The overwhelming power of European nations came to determine the process of medical reform clearly necessitated by the recent epidemics. The Muslim authorities intended European medical knowledge to fit within and to strengthen the indigenous power structure. But this was not to be the case.

Chapter 3

Cholera, typhus, and economic collapse, 1858–70

In the 1860s economic, political, social, and ecological crises ricocheted off one another in ominous succession. In the past Tunisia had weathered epidemics but this time new outbreaks of diseases in the context of the existing economic imbalance resulted in permanent damage to the established political order.

The weakness of the economy was exacerbated by new, European-imposed laws that removed the few remaining protections available to Tunisian commercial enterprises. Despite Muhammad Bey's conservatism, European interests in 1857 had induced him to promulgate a new charter, the *'ahd al-aman* (Fundamental Pact). The pact was essentially a bill of rights that was to become the basis of the 1860 constitution. Written by the French consul and rewritten by Bin Diyaf, the document gave Europeans the right to own land, to establish factories, and to practice free commerce. It abolished all legal protection for local products and industries. Rural qadis yielded their customary authority to newly created central criminal and commercial tribunals patterned after those of French civil law. Europeans were henceforth subject to local law, which was rewritten to give equal rights to all religions and nationalities. The consuls retained their extraterritorial rights, however, and continued to grant asylum not only to their conationals but also to Tunisians they chose to protect. The laws were adaptations of the Hatti Humayun and Hatti Sharif (tanzimat) Ottoman reform laws. Muhammad Bey ceremonially signed the pact, encouraged by the presence of a squadron of French and British warships moored off Tunis and Malta.[1]

The pact facilitated European investment, and the 1860s opened with a burst of economic activity. The decade closed with the Tunisian economy in shambles and under foreign management. Developmental projects led directly to the accumulation of a large public debt. European entrepreneurs had convinced the ruler Muhammad al-Sadiq Bey (1859–82) of the value of paved roads, railways, ferries, enlarged docks, telegraph lines, and aqueducts. He awarded concessions to various European companies to undertake projects intended to develop the economy and to make it more competitive on the world market. But the projects seldom showed a profit and losses were incurred by the bey, who had borrowed money to finance them. Bin Diyaf, for example, observed that the telegraph lines were useful in Europe, where the rural areas were heavily populated, but in the region between Tunis and Algeria there were no buildings where the lines could be hung, necessitating additional expenditure for poles. Also, the lines were easily cut by Bedouins, who resented the encroachment on their territories. The lines proved a convenience only to the French, who needed to communicate with their Algerian territories and with the ports of Tunisia, to which other lines were subsequently extended.[2]

Between 1860 and 1862 an annual average of 24 million francs was exchanged in the port of Tunis, a two-fold increase over yearly totals of the late 1840s. France, Italy, and England controlled 92 percent of the commercial exchange. But the value of exports equaled only 53 percent of the value of imports. Most of the exports were cereals and olive oil, whereas most of the imports were manufactured goods such as weapons, silks, linens, and cotton and wool textiles – goods that had been made locally and exported in the eighteenth century.[3]

The expansion of trade and the rapid integration of Tunisia into the European-dominated market masked a growing debt to local creditors which in 1860 stood at 19 million piasters (12 million francs). This slightly exceeded the average gross national product. In 1863 the first foreign loan was contracted with a prominent French banking house. The loan was for 39 million francs, which would amount to 65 million during the fifteen years of the repayment period. To repay the loan, the government guaranteed the entire annual *majba* (head tax) of 36 piasters levied since 1856, which was estimated at 5 million piasters. But only 30 million of the borrowed sum actually reached the treasury because of the habitual commissions, payments, and outright embezzlements by Tunisian and European agents, and the 30 million piasters disappeared within the year in payment of the local public debts and for public works.[4] By the end of 1863 it seemed that more money would not be forthcoming in the form of new loans, yet creditors were again demanding repayment.

There seemed to be no alternative but to raise taxes. They were already excessive and thoroughly resented by the populace, the vast majority of whom were dependent on agriculture. Incomes were low and disaster threatened when there was too much or too little rain or when epidemics or locusts struck. It was this subsistence sector that was being forced to support the new projects and fiscal policies of the commercial–political elite.[5]

In 1864 the government decided to double the head tax. The immediate decision throughout Tunisia was to resist. Peasants, nomadic and seminomadic tribesmen, and townspeople joined in spontaneous armed resistance, which spread during the spring and summer of 1864. Government troops put down the revolt with great difficulty. The new head tax finally was abolished and amnesty proclaimed. The amnesty was violated, however, and rebel towns were pillaged by the government because of their actions. About 100 million piasters were extorted as indemnity. Many people were forced to take out loans at usurious interest rates of 40 to 100 percent to pay their fines and were thus forced into debt for years to come.[6]

During the 1864 revolt, land had not been cultivated, and in the repression, capital for replanting was seized. A spiral of crises followed. In 1865 rains were too heavy in some areas, while in the wheat-growing northwest a long drought continued. The result was widespread famine which worsened toward the end of 1865. At the beginning of 1866 Bayram al-Khamis provided a personal account of the misery which followed the repression and famine:

...the villages, tribes, and towns were left with nothing. Poverty was everywhere and those who had the least bit of food were hiding it and sending their women to collect grass in the fields or to search for the roots of trees for food. One of the Drid tribe mentioned that he had sent his women, who knew nothing of the desert, to bring roots of *tirfas* [truffle] and to put it outside his house so that the *'amil*'s [district officer's] guards would see it and think that he had nothing. In the evening, he would cook his wheat without milling so that the noise would not be heard, and people would not know that he had money.[7]

The indemnities exacted after the 1864 revolt offered the government a temporary reprive from defaulting on loan payments. The harvests of 1864–5 had been exceptionally meager. The drought continued and there was little likelihood that further plunder of the country's resources would yield sufficient revenue. Nevertheless, the government again sent the mahalla toward the western region. According to Bin Diyaf, the people of Tunis were amazed at the government's audacity as the tribes were already reduced to eating wild roots and religiously forbidden foods such as carrion.[8] The armed government troops accompanying the expedition forced the western tribes to pay. The tribesmen had to sell the last of their grain to pay the tax, leaving none to replant the following year. In the words of Bin Diyaf, 'they started selling their horses.... Their God made them perish through cold and hunger because there were no more plants to eat.' Normally, the tribespeople periodically visited the regional markets to sell their livestock, but now 'their caravans started coming and going with skin and bones to sell. The market places of the rural districts were almost restricted to selling skin and bones, dead animals, and rags of the poor who lay dead on the ground.' The final disaster came when they were 'forced to sell their tents and went to live with their children under the sky, left to the cold and heat'.[9] Bin Diyaf adds that there were many deaths among the people who were weakened and without adequate food or shelter. The destitute people then began converging on the capital city expecting that the ruler would offer them public assistance.

All the government received from its mahalla expedition to the west and south was 180,000 piasters and 300,000 piasters, respectively, far short of the expected four million that had already been promised to European creditors.[10] To make matters worse, the olive crop of 1866 had been sold in advance to European merchants and when the crop failed, the creditors again expected the government to make up the difference, with interest. In June 1866 the government defaulted on its loan payments and there was another attempt to raise money by increasing taxes. This time a tax on olive trees was levied, but in Cap Bon, a prosperous region that had escaped the worst effects of the rebellion and drought, growers found revenues from the successful crop of 1866 not enough to pay the new tax. The owners were forced to make up the difference from their own funds and many had to contract loans at the usual usurious interest rates charged by rural creditors. The following year the owners saw no point in taking care of their trees, production further declined, and 'the prisons weren't large enough for all the owners, and the trees of the Cap Bon were lost because of this tax.... The people threw up their hands and left things to God.'[11]

In Tunis people were dying of hunger in the streets, and the inhabitants there wearied of beggars who went from house to house asking for food.[12] Many of the impoverished were members of defeated tribes, made destitute by the indemnities and taxes. Others were members of the European communities. The vast majority of Europeans lived in squalor, having come to Tunis for lack of work in their native Sicily or Malta. The European quarters were crowded and dirty and, like the indigenous neighborhoods, were to become foyers for epidemic diseases:

At Tunis, as at Sousse and Sfax, the European quarter extended from the lower part of the native city. Drains open to the sky collected rain water and refuse from the upper quarters. The drains ran into a blackish, smelly mire which transformed all the streets into marshes. Household garbage was tossed freely; in Tunis, pigs by the hundreds vagabonded at will, rooting in the drains and the piles of rubbish.[13]

The stage for the next crisis was set.

Cholera, 1867, aftermath of revolution

In 1867 the Sanitary Council had been in existence for more than a generation. Tunis was in contact with the International Sanitary Commission in Istanbul, its new government newspaper, *Ra'id al-tunisi*, printed international quarantining regulations, and its new telegraph lines carried news of outbreaks of communicable diseases in various ports of the Mediterranean.[14] There were quarantine officials stationed throughout the country and Muslim and European functionaries were instructed to report disease outbreaks to the authorities in Tunis. The bankrupt government, however, was to prove less concerned with disease prevention than in previous decades and the Sanitary Council and *ad hoc* committees played a more active role. To many, the government as a result appeared to have abandoned its traditional responsibilities of providing relief and thereby to have relinquished one of the bases of its political legitimacy. But the government had been rendered ineffective not by the epidemics but by the consequences of the European economic expansion.

At the first news of cholera in Alexandria, efforts to police the coasts of Tunisia were increased. Rustam, the Mamluk minister of the interior, then ordered the commanding officer of the A'rad (southern) region and all port authorities to refuse entry to ships from Egypt. But the orders proved difficult as ever to implement.[15]

It was nearly impossible to stop all communication with outside regions and thus to prevent any contact with the disease, but diligent efforts to carry out the recommendations of the Sanitary Council continued. One problem, for example, concerned the surveillance of fishing vessels. In August 1865 the 'amil of Bizerte complained to Mustafa, the prime minister, that coral-fishing boats from Algeria were getting their food from caches they had hidden in secluded beaches.[16] Another difficulty involved the control of smuggling. Tunisians, Maltese, and Sicilians were engaged in an active trade in contraband that had increased in the 1860s with illegal arms purchases used in the 1864 insurrection and with the export of overtaxed crops.

Cholera, transmitted through water contaminated by infected individuals, was apparently brought into Tunisia from Sicily by way of the illegal trade. It first appeared in a small coastal town, between Tunis and Bizerte, which was a center for smuggling from Sicily, where the disease was then raging. This town, Qal'at al-Andalus,[17] was stricken with an epidemic in April 1867. When news of the outbreak reached Tunis, two doctors, Schembri and Cotton, were sent to the town to make a report.[18] On 19 April an epidemic of cholera was announced in Qal'at al-Andalus.[19]

The 'amil of Bizerte immediately went to the town to evaluate the conditions. According to his report, he assembled the people and asked them about their situation. They replied that the disease was indeed raging and that twenty persons had died since the *'id*, a yearly feast. The victims included six men, seven women, and seven children. Another fifty, mostly children, were still sick and were suffering from 'pain in the heart and sides, a need to drink much water, vomiting and diarrhea, with many of the stricken dying within twenty-four hours of the onset of symptoms'.[20] This description of the symptoms left little doubt that the disease was cholera.

A week later the shaykh of the village wrote to the military command in Tunis asking for help. In his letter he described the situation of his people:

...we are in hardship from hunger and the calamity. Some of the people are stealing from each other and others are helping one another. All of the Spanish [the inhabitants of Qal'at al-Andalus] have come to a standstill. The country is having the weather of summertime. There are no plants, no beans, barley, wheat, or grasses. There is nothing for the animals to eat. The people are flocking to us every day. They want us to tell you about our problem so that you will do something for us.[21]

Relief was apparently not sent, though a cordon was placed around the town. Fortunately, the epidemic ceased as abruptly as it had begun, and on 9 May Drs Nachtigal[22] and Prats, who had been sent from the capital to report on the situation, declared the town cholera-free.[23] The cordon was maintained until the first week in June, despite the pleading of the shaykh to the military command that the disease had passed and that the cordon was 'very trying'.[24]

The efforts to contain the epidemic were not successful, and the disease broke out in Bizerte in mid-May. By the end of May regular reports of the sickness were being sent to Rustam, the minister of the interior, from the *khalifa* (provincial governor).[25] At first he was optimistic that the disease would subside. He also felt that the heat wave and famine were ending since it was raining slightly, and new vegetables and cereals were expected.[26] But by the third week of June, it was clear that the disease was not abating.

Dr Honoré They, a French doctor who had been sent to Bizerte, telegraphed a report to N. Vignale, the Italian *bash tabib* (head doctor) in Tunis.[27] In the report They said he was well received by the 'amil of Bizerte. He may have heard of the hostility that greeted Mancel in the same town in 1850, when its inhabitants suspected him of causing the disease and forced him to leave the town for fear of his life. Dr They immediately learned from the 'amil that during the previous twenty-five days, five hundred Muslims, fifty Jews, and five Christians had perished and that another five hundred Muslims had fled the town. Since the total population of Bizerte was about ten thousand, the extent of the calamity was very serious.

They proceeded to visit as many of the sick as possible and had a very difficult time, though he expressed guarded confidence in his medical ability:

Until now, my day's work is not done. It is impossible for me to visit all the sick in one day, especially in the *impasses* [narrow streets and blind alleys] where the Muslims live. I am doing all I can, without delay in work, to give assistance. In five days, I visited 268 persons sick with cholera. Many call me when cure is of no use, but when people of the city call me in the beginning of the sickness, it doesn't get worse, God willing....[28]

The doctor noted that the Muslim and Jewish communities responded differently to his services: 'Many Muslims want neither the doctor nor medicine, but as for the Jews, they call the doctor right away.' Some Muslims did seek his aid, as shown by his comment that even after the disease had ceased in the Jewish quarter: 'I am still running night and day to help the sick all twenty-four hours. I sleep only four hours. There is no time for me to write this report to you....'

To emphasize the miserable conditions under which he was practicing, They elaborated on the situation that existed in the main square of town: 'Even while I write you this report, a large number of inhabitants are milling in the center of town, calling upon God to help them. I have seen things here which tear the heart out – people are expiring in the impasses and in the saqifa of the mosque of Sidi al-Bahri.'[29]

He astutely observed that it was a combination of cholera and famine that had stricken the region: 'The people die of the calamity and from hunger. There are houses in which four or five have died and this is still continuing.... Hunger, upset, and lack of organization are [contributing] causes of this death and peril.' He complained that the whole madina and the interior streets were in an unsanitary condition. Bad meat was being offered for sale and people were forced to buy it. He said the Muslims were eating too many cucumbers, tomatoes, melons, and bad fruits. It seems that the doctor's concern was justified since poor sanitation contributes to cholera epidemics, and every summer Tunisia suffered from outbreaks of 'summer fever', caused by excessive consumption of unripe fruit.

Dr They made no mention of any indigenous practitioners in the town and complained that he was all alone with no assistance other than that of two of the Sisters of Saint Joseph. He concluded his letter with a note that he would be willing to leave the town to its own devices if so ordered by Vignale.[30]

In the same week that They sent his telegram, the khalifa of Bizerte wrote to Rustam reporting that 178 persons had died during the week in the region of Bizerte and that more than twenty were still dying per day. He had heard that an assistant was being sent and he thanked Rustam in advance. In a postscript he added that seventy persons had died in Ras Jabal.[31] Perhaps those fleeing Bizerte had brought the disease with them to the surrounding areas.

The letters suggest the extent of the disruption of normal life. This description is corroborated by mortality statistics. In a final report the khalifa reported that a total of eleven hundred had died in Bizerte and four hundred in Ras Jabal, or about 10 percent of the population in each case. He said that people were terrorized and all movement had stopped during the epidemic. But people were back at work in mid-July and the disease had disappeared in the region by the end of the month.[32]

On 23 May 1867 the mahalla under the command of Ahmad Zarruq left for the A'rad to the south going by way of the Sahel.[33] Some of the officers and troops fell sick *en route*. A few days later, on the first of June, cholera broke out among the inhabitants of Sousse.[34] Panic followed as groups of Europeans scrambled to board a steamship bound for Livorno. A few people in prison for debts to these creditors were set free for the duration of the epidemic.[35]

Rustam sent orders to the khalifa of Sousse telling him to see that the streets were cleaned and that the sick were forcibly isolated on the outskirts of town. The khalifa responded that the shaykhs of the town found it impossible to remove those who fell sick from their households, as their families would not allow them to be carried out. He added that the families would be very much afflicted if they could not care for their sick at home. The consul general of Italy in Sousse also telegraphed the prime minister protesting the order, which, he said, would 'cause the gravest disorders among the population which had been badly decimated by the disease'. He asked that the bey be informed of the order.[36]

A few days after the outbreak in Sousse, cholera appeared in nearby Monastir, where it took a similar course. Debtors were let out of prison and orders were sent to isolate the risk. Incense was to be burned in the rooms where deaths had occurred, and the rooms were to be whitewashed in order to purify them. The khalifa of Monastir selected the *zawiya* (small mosque and hospice) of Sidi Muhammad al-Mazari for the isolation of the sick, but again the shaykhs of the city could not force people to let their sick be taken away.[37]

Daily reports were sent as required and mortality reports were grouped into divisions of Muslims, Jews, and Christians. During June and July 1867 a total of about fifteen hundred perished in the region of Sousse and Monastir according to these reports.[38]

Many Europeans were convinced that Muslims assumed a passive fatalistic attitude toward epidemics. The people of unaffected Mahdiya and Sfax, however, placed cordons around their city boundaries to prevent persons from Sousse, Monastir, and the surrounding towns, where cholera was raging, from entering their territories. In Mahdiya numerous complaints had been made to the khalifa against families who were fleeing there from Sousse. The cordon was ungenerously set up to prevent further arrivals.[39] In Sfax the cordon was placed around the city to prevent contact with the army of the tax-gathering expedition which was then camped nearby.[40] Cholera was more clearly contagious than plague and during the 1867 epidemic all controversy over protection by quarantine seems to have ceased.

During the famine that preceded the epidemic government troops had been sent to the Beja region to stop marauding nomads who had been pillaging granaries. The tribespeople had been destitute since the 1864 rebellion and many had already died of starvation.[41] Reinforcements had been sent out at the beginning of June, and these troops had stopped a few days in Bizerte. A few cases of cholera broke out among them while they were *en route* to Beja, and within a few days of their passing the disease was raging in the entire region.[42]

In Tunis the government and European inhabitants feared the pillaging of government granaries would erupt into an uprising on the scale of the 1864 insurrection. There had been threatening disturbances in several cities in the Sahel and among the tribes of the Djerid. But the epidemic undermined further efforts at resistance to government policy. The 'amil of Bizerte in fact wrote with relief that the sickness had disciplined the nomads into obedience because they were preoccupied with caring for their sick.[43]

Unfortunately, there are no mortality statistics for the western region, probably because the telegraph line was not working. The line was repeatedly cut by nomads, who saw it as an unwelcome intrusion into their territories. By all reports mortality was at least as high as during the 1849 epidemic. Bin Diyaf reported in his account that the population of Beja was almost annihilated.[44]

By July the disease was raging through the southern region of the Djerid, in the oases of Tozeur and Nafta, and in the city of Gafsa. The first week of July the 'amil of the Djerid reported by letter that the disease had taken four hundred people, of whom thirty were from the army, and

73

that the disease was still spreading.[45] He added that he had organized a funeral procession for the dead from among the army personnel and had arranged to give money to the poor.

The majority of the population in the southern desert region was nomadic, and the 'amil complained that the Farashish tribe had camped around the oases and was making trouble: 'They enter the gardens and live in small houses and go asking for alms. The people of the Djerid do not have enough for them so they are using their strength and are stealing. The people are thinking of forcing them out.'[46] In later reports the 'amil wrote that the nomads and people of the oases were starving and eating unripe dates. Trees and plants were without irrigation as people were too sick to take care of them. He estimated that at least three hundred had died from the cholera epidemic in the oases and that more than one thousand had perished in Gafsa, twelve hundred in Tozeur, and two thousand in Nafta.[47]

The island of Djerba was cordoned off with a twenty-one-day quarantine placed on all incoming ships. This was a great hardship for the island's people since they were already suffering from the famine. On 16 July the shaykhs of the island sent a letter to the sahib al-taba' informing him that two ships full of wheat and barley had arrived from Libya. Although their patents were marked 'foul' (meaning cholera had been present at the port of origin), the ships were accepted by the quarantine officials, who then sent for the notables of the famine-stricken island. A council meeting was held concerning the acceptance of the much-needed provisions. After heated discussion, a decision was made to accept the ships, and the cereals were unloaded and aired. The shaykhs based their decision on the fact that 'hunger was worse than the sickness'. The ships and their passengers were sent away after the grain was unloaded.[48]

For many months people had been going to Tunis from the famished rural areas. The already congested poorer quarters and the lack of hygiene made the city's environment ideal for the spread of epidemic disease. The drains serving the crowded city were shallow open-air drains constructed of clay brick. The wells and cisterns were easily contaminated by seepage from these drains and from the uncollected refuse in the streets.[49]

The Sanitary Council acknowledged the danger and made repeated recommendations for better sanitation and quarantine precautions.[50] Finally, a cordon was placed at Hammam Lif to the south of the city to prevent the sick from entering Tunis. Travelers from Bizerte were also checked for illness but the disease had already broken out among the troops in Tunis. The cordons served only to detain travelers temporarily. There was little hope that the city would be spared a general outbreak of cholera. As cases of the disease increased among the civilians of Tunis, the Sanitary Council called a meeting with doctors of the city. After deliberation, an epidemic in the city of Tunis was announced.[51]

In the words of one of the doctors, 'fear spread like a cold wave throughout the city'.[52] Those who could fled, the wealthy Europeans leaving first. Following its usual course, the disease first spread in the Jewish quarter and then to the rest of the city. By the third week of June, deaths numbered a hundred and fifty per day.[53] Bayram al-Khamis described the situation in Tunis in 1867:

Their poverty, misery, and oppression were not enough. Hunger, drought, and famine overtook them and the lack of capital to cultivate the land caused the urban population to share their predicament as their fortune was linked to that of the rural area. Groups of people flocked to the capital and to the cities from all directions. Only a few were to reach the city because of the malignant fever which struck them. The sickness decimated the people and their cadavers remained in the desert for the beasts of prey.[54]

The maristan was exceedingly crowded during the epidemic with the poor seeking refuge there. Like the emergency hospitals, it cannot have served more than a few dozen people at a time though it remained in very active use. In the 1860s the hospital was still located in the same two-story building originally allocated for the purpose in 1662. During the 1867 cholera epidemic, a prominent Italian doctor, Mugnaini, visited the maristan to consult with patients there in his efforts to disprove other doctors' diagnoses of a contagious epidemic.[55] The responsibility for medical care and general public assistance was left to private persons. A group of notables (prominent townspeople) was organized by Husayn Sharif[56] to help the destitute by giving them money for food and shelter. As the disease worsened, these notables repeatedly asked the government for help, which was not forthcoming. Bin Diyaf observed that at the time of greatest difficulty, Mustafa Khaznadar, the Mamluk treasurer, who had retained contact with his native Greece, sent ten thousand riyals from the state treasury to two Greek nephews he was educating in Paris.[57]

French and Jewish merchants organized another group which collected money and set up a temporary hospital at the entrance of Bab al-Bahr, with doctors and twenty workers to care for the sick among the poor of all denominations. Independently of the government they provided food and medicine with the money collected and sent a doctor and medicine to those unable to go to Bab al-Bahr.[58]

While the private charities of Husayn Sharif and the merchants provided for the needy of all religions and nationalities, other groups were organized for the aid of their conationals alone. In a report to the

Foreign Office a British consular official wrote that while there was a much greater panic than during the previous epidemic and many wealthy Europeans had left the country, the British had been foremost among those who had remained in donating funds to help their countrymen. He added that the government of Malta had telegraphed one hundred pounds to help Maltese who might be stricken with the disease.[59]

An account by Ferrini, an Italian doctor, mentioned a relief committee organized from among the membership of an Italian workers' organization which was headed by one Angelo Blanch. This group set up a hospital staffed with young Italian volunteers from among the well-to-do families and 'honest workmen'.[60] Ferrini could not resist including an evaluation of his colleagues' behavior during the cholera epidemic: 'The doctors, with the exception of one, the softness of whose guts suggested to him to close himself in a quarantine of his own house, threw themselves fully into their duty, giving to all without distinction of any nationality, any hour of the day, the necessary care. Not only the doctors but also the pharmacists did more than their duty in providing for the poor sick with free medicine.'

The great majority of the people were, however, left to care for themselves, with the aid of indigenous doctors and the traditional remedies such as honey and olive oil. This was not necessarily unfortunate. Remedies used by European doctors had not greatly improved since previous epidemics, though bleeding to remove excess blood was less frequently performed. Mugnaini recommended against the use of laxatives and suggested a mixture of poppy seeds and laudanum taken orally or by enema. His prescription had, he said, 'succeeded in thousands of cases'. Other remedies in common use by the European doctors were: coffee, calomine, opiates, laudanum, and sodium and magnesium sulfates. None of these medicines was effective in curing cholera though they may have served to ameliorate gastrointestinal symptoms.[61]

Sadiq Bey was still clinging to his palace as the famished and sick demanded assistance and creditors clamored to be repaid. There had been almost no revenues collected during 1866 and the epidemic of 1867 had worsened the financial situation of Tunisia. A British consular official summarized the situation:

The visitation of the present epidemic is the most deplorable calamity that could have befallen [Tunisia] at a moment when the government on the one hand is labouring under financial difficulties and embarrassments, thereby paralysing its action even to the collection of Public Revenues, and on the other, the distress and misery that exists throughout the Regency owing to the failure of the crops, combined with the stagnation of trade and the suspension of all work and occupation, have greatly aggravated the suffering that is at present felt by the entire population.[62]

This situation continued throughout the summer months. While the city attempted to care for its sick and impoverished inhabitants (still without governmental assistance), the Sanitary Council continued to meet. Its members debated the length of quarantine to be imposed on ships coming from ports infected with cholera, though this could hardly have made any difference at this point. They also discussed the proper burial of corpses as a way of containing the disease for it was still widely believed that fumes from decomposing matter caused the disease.[63]

Not surprisingly, in view of the conditions in the city, little was done to implement the council's recommendations. Toward the end of August, however, it was clear that the disease was abating. Questionnaires were sent to nine of the city's doctors asking them to report on the extent of the disease. On 3 September 1867 the Sanitary Council met to discuss the responses, and on the basis of the results the epidemic was officially declared over. Only a few cases had been seen in nearly a month and they were seemingly isolated ones. The question of issuing clean or foul patents to ships leaving La Goulette was put to the council and the members present voted unanimously to issue clean patents.[64] On 19 October the *Ra'id al-tunisi* carried an open letter from the bey to Vignale, his personal physician, asking him to thank the doctors of the capital who had worked hard during the epidemic.[65] Other than this brief word, the government newspaper had scarcely mentioned the crisis. But the cholera epidemic was not forgotten; it became known as *bu shalal* (in Tunisian colloquial Arabic, 'severe dysentery'). The year 1284 AH/1867 AD was subsequently referred to as 'the year of bu shalal'.[66]

In September the harvest was much below expectation. And with winter approaching, the unhappy inhabitants still had to face months of hunger and cold.[67] In November a second flood of Bedouins arrived in Tunis in hope of public assistance. Like the earlier arrivals, they had sold their food stores, livestock, and tents and began camping in the streets of the capital with the rest of the impoverished immigrants.[68] When the severe winter arrived, the indigent crowded into makeshift shelters. Bin Diyaf provided an eyewitness description of the city and of the maristan, which was but a short distance from his residence: 'Every morning, coffins were seen going back and forth from the maristan. The number dying per day rose to about a hundred. The treasury was exhausted from burying them and from paying for the shrouds. The city was reeking from rotting corpses and refuse. People were falling sick in the alleys. The doctors cautioned against this and warned that another [epidemic] sickness would come and it did.'[69]

Typhus, 1868, prelude to bankruptcy

The doctors feared an outbreak of plague, but typhus broke out instead. The milling crowds, wearing heavy woolen *burnuses* (hooded cloaks) against the winter cold, were ideal candidates for an epidemic of typhus, a lice-borne disease that typically strikes refugees living in unsanitary conditions.

Typhus first appeared toward the end of 1867; an epidemic was officially announced on 12 February 1868.[70] The disease did not have the shock value of cholera as its symptoms were not as unfamiliar or dramatic, but it was just as deadly. Since it was not among the diseases that were considered to travel from port to port, typhus was not subject to quarantine and there are consequently fewer government records of its progress.

As usual the bey was besieged by pleas to do something about the situation. Werry, vice president of the Sanitary Council, wrote to Mustafa Khaznadar asking him to encourage the bey to take steps to alleviate the consequences of the new epidemic. He said that he felt it his duty to inform the minister of the numerous corpses left unburied in the streets of the city. Echoing other accounts, he reminded Mustafa that 'the misery is great this year. A frightful famine is decimating the Arab populations. A rigorous cold ordinarily unknown in these regions has joined the scourge and daily carries off numerous victims.'[71] Basing his argument on the miasma theory of disease transmission, he informed the minister that a 'perturbation of the vital elements of the atmosphere which has already produced terrible effects, has resulted from rotting corpses and menaces us with the most frightful of calamities – the plague! Typhus already reigns in Tunis in a frightful manner. My particular information from the most distinguished doctors of the country makes me believe that at the first heat, the evil germs will transmute in a proportion which will be impossible to stop and in this case, very difficult to combat.' Werry further asked that the bey be urged to take measures to combat the scourge which menaced them all, Arabs and Europeans alike.[72]

But Mustafa's replies were evasive and again included the statements 'other nations suffer too' and 'it is the will of God'. Both the Arabic and the European accounts mention with bitterness these remarks to the Sanitary Council. Citing his lack of interest as evidence of the government's indifference, the Sanitary Council announced that it intended to act without official sanction and to exceed its status as an advisory council.

On 12 February 1868 the council issued orders for the creation of an *ad hoc* Sanitary Police to clean the streets of Tunis on a daily basis. The council asked the government to give an order for the general cleaning of the city, after which committees formed from each quarter were to be charged with cleaning their own streets. The European inhabitants of Tunis were becoming more independent of the central government. On 23 February the new Sanitary Police Committee was formed under the first article of the Municipal Police Corps, which had been established as part of the Municipal Council of 1858.[73]

The Sanitary Council announced a new list of public health rules. The rules were concerned with the removal to Muhammadiya of mendicant Bedouins from the city of Tunis, with the disposal of both animal and human corpses, and with the isolation and care of the sick. The council ruled that lime be thrown on the cadavers and that they be buried at least two meters below the surface. It called for the evacuation of prisons and barracks and the whitewashing of their walls, the clearing away of skin and bones of animals, and the draining of mires.[74]

After these orders were issued, the acrimonious tone of the correspondence between the Sanitary Council and the government increased. The council informed the minister that his statement that 'misery exists in other countries' was not satisfactory because in other countries 'governments do all they can to fight against the misery [of epidemic disease]'.[75] The council went on to inform Mustafa that although it did not doubt the benevolent intentions of His Majesty, the orders had not been satisfactorily executed. The goverment was further informed that the Sanitary Council was 'composed of accredited consuls of foreign powers' and with that authority had decided to form an *ad hoc* committee under the presidency of G. Harris Heap, the consul general of the United States. The committee would clean and make healthy that part of the city inhabited by Europeans. The consuls had, in effect, instituted their own 'public health service' without sanction from the bey.[76]

This was the first example of independent political action taken by Europeans as a reaction to the inaction of the beylical government. At one point Richard Wood had even suggested forcing the bey to take measures to clean the rue des Maltais, which bordered the Jewish quarter, where the sickness was especially severe. At one meeting of the council, the condition of the street was described in lurid detail. One member of the committee who had walked through the hara and then the rue des Maltais 'wondered not why the epidemic raged with vigor among the Jewish population but why it was not more severe'.[77]

The crisis continued. As typhus spread, Mustafa Khaznadar was pressured by the Sanitary Council into ratifying the public health program.[78] City facilities to manage such an epidemic were clearly inadequate. Bin Diyaf mentions severe overcrowding in the maristan with coffins daily carried out to the Jalaz cemetery as in the cholera epidemic.[79] Finally, a locale outside the city was prepared for the isolation of the sick. A singularly poor choice, it was an unused *ma'sr al-zaytun* (building where olive oil was pressed) and was dark, dank, and poorly ventilated.[80]

The council took advantage of its victory and issued more rules concerning the disposal of garbage, the proper management of fruit and vegetable shops, the flow of traffic, the numbering of carts and commercial taxis, the proper butchering of meat, and the nomination of guards for Tunis and the villages around it. Taxes were imposed for the new services. But two months later the council was still complaining about the state of sanitation in the city.[81]

As the sickness persisted, Khaznadar persuaded the bey to turn again to the wealthy notables. Their wealth was assessed and the extorted funds channeled through the organization of Husayn Sharif.[82] The bey gave fifteen thousand riyals, Mustafa Khaznadar contributed seven thousand (as compared with the ten thousand he had sent to his nephews), and each of the notables, five thousand. Qa'id Nassim Samama, a Jewish official who, like Bin 'Ayad, had absconded with at least a hundred thousand riyals from the treasury in 1864 in addition to other funds, sent twenty-five thousand riyals for the relief of the Jewish community. Bayram al-Khamis expressed disgust with the bey, who had given only fifteen thousand riyals from the public treasury. But he reflected that perhaps the bey was not to blame as he had insisted that he was himself in financial straits. Bayram had heard that the bey had instructed the keeper of the *ma'mal al-khubz* (bakery) to send bread for his family, as they were unable to obtain any. Bayram was also disgusted with Khaznadar, who had not done more to help, and disapprovingly cited his statement that 'other nations suffered too'.[83]

During the worst days of the crisis Bayram wrote a letter to a friend describing the times through which he was living: 'If you could come and see our condition, you would be filled with terror and you would try to flee, to escape from wild wolves and sly foxes, which chase people and scatter men escaping from grasping snakes which crave for money. What a miserable state for anyone who has to stay in this place!'[84] His own reaction, as a member of the wealthy elite, was to try to leave, but he was hindered by his landholdings and family:

The state is collapsing and is on its way to deterioration or extinction. Men are shaken to their foundations. People are dying very young, there is no hope for anyone. Recovery seems almost impossible. . . . I swear by the Prophet Muhammad that I tried several times to leave the country but I was bound to it by my condition and by my family. . . . I offered my property for sale and tried to 'pull up my tent pegs' but I didn't find anyone to buy it.[85]

Bayram concluded by describing the situation in the streets, where the destitute were milling:

People are perplexed. They cannot take a decision. They are starving to the extent that they would eat iron if it was available and even ask for more. You see the people drunk but they are not drunk. This is the result of God's curse and torture. On the roads you hear groans and at every door, people are shouting out of anger. Tumult at the market prevails. The crowd is desperate, people are swarming and pushing. . . .[86]

A last attempt at rebellion was again made by the western tribes when a younger brother of the bey arrived there to revive the 1864 attempt. He failed and was captured by the authorities and died in prison. Notables of the region said the attempt failed because 'the epidemic had extinguished the fire of revolt as people were preoccupied with caring for the sick and dying'.[87]

Social and economic consequences of the 1867–8 epidemics

Bin Diyaf gloomily wondered whether 'one-half of the population had perished, or perhaps two-thirds, with one-third remaining'.[88] A work stoppage during summer 1867 had caused the smallest revenue collection of the decade. Shares of Tunisian obligations on the Paris stock exchange plunged to their lowest levels of the decade during the months of epidemic disease.[89]

For the first time, the French consul spoke of military occupation to ensure repayment of loans. In October 1867 Napoleon III had presided over a secret meeting of a council of ministers during which it was decided to send an expedition of eight thousand men to occupy the port of Tunis. French functionaries stationed in Tunisian ports were to oversee the collection of custom duties and taxes which were to be used to repay French creditors. The chargé d'affaires in Tunis informed the emperor that 'the Regency of Tunis was at the disposal of any government that considered it in their interest to take possession of it. . . .'[90] Because of the civil war in Rome to which French troops were committed, the plan had to be postponed. It was not abandoned entirely.

Meanwhile, Italy and England voiced their resentment of France's assumption of a special protective role in Tunisia, and after months of negotiation the three nations reached an agreement on the joint management of Tunisian finances. In 1869 the International Financial Commission was established to reorganize Tunisia's economy and to pay the debt as a first priority.[91]

The beylical government had been rendered incapable of taking action against the epidemics. The bankrupt government could no longer manage its paternal role in providing charities. The 'ulama' were not heard from as mediators or advisers in the epidemics of the 1860s. Charities were organized by European and Muslim *ad hoc* committees with considerable local powers. Did the traditional leadership's failure to cope with the 1867–8 cholera and typhus epidemics discredit it in the popular eye, as McNeill suggested, leading to acceptance of Western medicine? Perhaps the leadership's failure to cope with the wider challenge of the European impact had discredited it. The insurrection of 1864 and subsequent manifestations of discontent were primarily protests against severely worsened economic conditions. The insurrectionists wanted to return to traditional ways since the European reforms seemed only to harm them. Medicine was one of the areas in which anti-European sentiments surfaced.

Again, the economic disruption was not caused solely by the epidemics. This time, however, the existing domestic and international crises combined with the panic, work stoppage, and loss of life resulting from cholera and typhus led to the first stage of foreign takeover. As is seen in Appendix C, at least 10,000 from Tunis alone, a city of about 150,000, had perished in the 1867–8 epidemics. This loss of life could not be overlooked by the leadership. But who was the leadership in the political or medical spheres?

The bey had proven unable to provide assistance and his minister, Khaznadar, had become a symbol of governmental impotence. Muslim and European communities had taken to running independent *ad hoc* public health boards. As will be shown in Chapter 4, European doctors had quietly taken over the licensing functions of the amin al-atibba' in the early 1860s. Following the epidemic, Tunisian reformers in effect took over the goverment and made medical reforms a central part of their programs. The Muslim reformers, the bey and his coterie, and Italian and French agents now tried to guide Tunisia's future in their respective interests. The victors of the struggle were to form new laws and institutions in the medical sector that became a justification of their presence in Tunisia and a basis of their political legitimacy.

Chapter 4

Colonization and collapse of Arab medical institutions

Throughout the years of the plague and cholera epidemics, Muslim doctors continued to serve the majority of the population. Most were unlicensed empirics who had learned their trade from apprenticeships or experience. Until the early 1860s, however, the amin al-atibba' continued to issue ijazas to applicants, usually in exchange for written proof of experience and a small fee. The amin continued in his role as head of the maristan, which remained the only Muslim hospital in Tunis. The authority of the Muslim amin diminished in the 1860s and 1870s until the last non-European-trained amin died in 1876. But the choice of medical systems had long become clear – European medicine was officially to prevail. The only questions were under whose authority and in what form. Were the reforms to take place under beylical authority or under a colonial government, and were the medical authorities to be European-trained Muslims or Europeans themselves? And if they were to be the latter, would they be Italian, British or French officials?

Transition from Muslim to European medical authority

The indigenous medical institutions continued to function until the middle of the nineteenth century. The bey's European doctor was still responsible only to the court while the Muslim amin al-atibba' or the bey himself was in charge of licensing the indigenous doctors. Ijazas are preserved in the government archives issued by Ahmad Bey in 1840 to indigenous doctors; the last one is dated 1861 and was issued by Muhammad al-Sadiq Bey.[1]

In the early 1860s, however, the ubiquitous Dr Lumbroso replaced the amin al-atibba' as medical licensor. Fig. 5 shows a typical medical ijaza issued in 1861, to al-Hajj b. 'Abd al-Karim al-Siba'i al-Maghribi.[2] The signature and handwriting indicate that the issuer was Muhammad bu 'Asida, the same individual who had renewed al-Kilani's certificate in 1855 (mentioned in Chapter 1). Also in 1861 an ijaza, this time written in Italian, was issued to 'Si el Hag Hosayn ben Haled el Kerim Esbahi

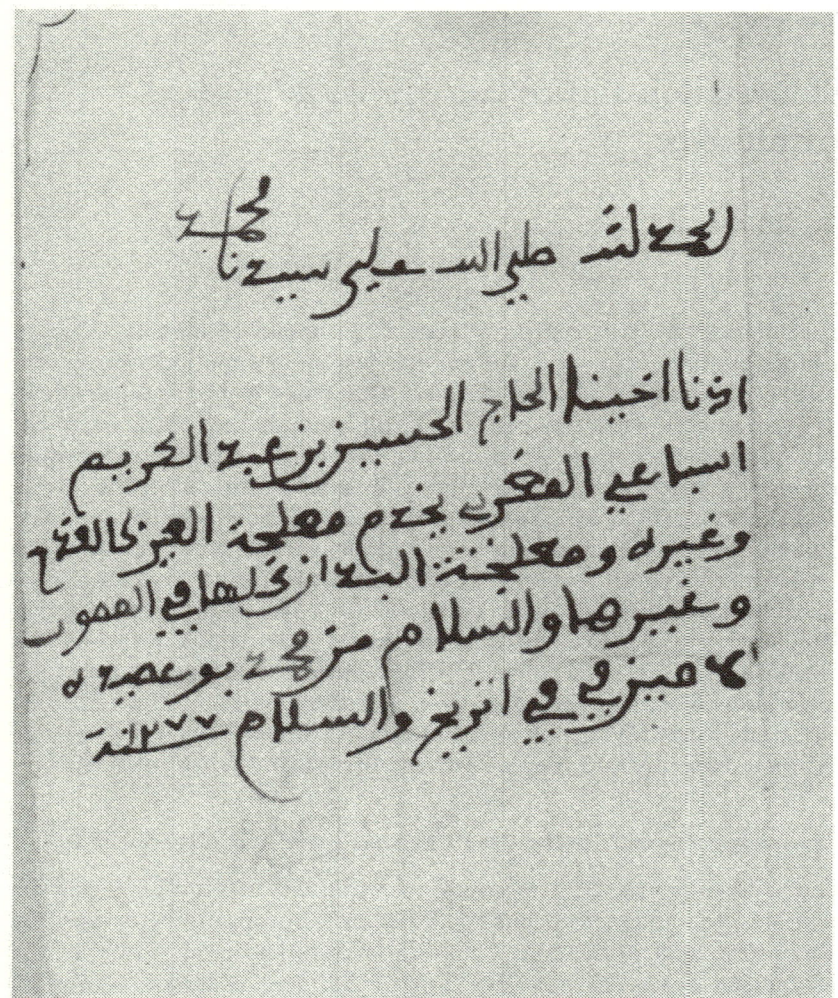

Fig. 5. Ijaza issued in 1861 to al-Hajj b. 'Abd al-Karim al-Siba'i al-Maghribi by Muhammad bu 'Asida

di Marrocco' to practice as 'Officiale Sanitario Empirico'.[3] The names indicate that the recipients were one and the same person. Evidently, doctors seeking licenses were now obliged to obtain verification from the bey's official physician, who had served as director of health since 1856. After this date, all ijazas on record were issued by the bey's European doctor, who now collected the fees formerly paid to the amin. Numerous copies of the licenses are preserved in the government archives.

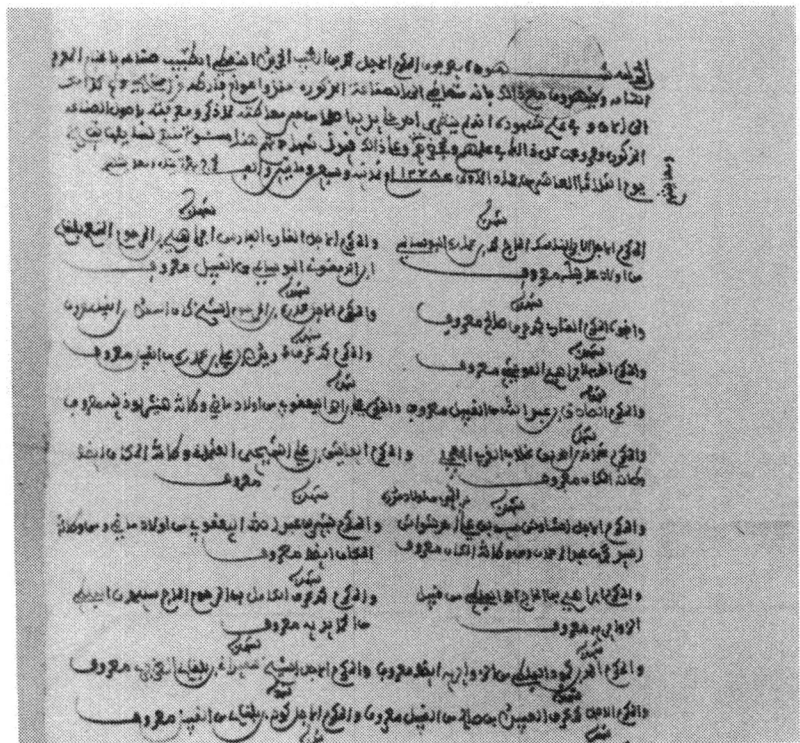

Fig. 6(a). Part of a petition testifying that al-Nafti has practiced medicine in the Djerid for years without harming anyone, signed by witnesses from the region (additional signatures follow)

In 1861, for example, Muhammad b. Tabib al-Jaridi al-Nafti had a document drawn up in his district near Beja. It stated that he had 'practiced medicine for several years without doing harm to his patients, and was a competent doctor'. The document was ratified by sixty witnesses from the region who signed their names to it. It was then ratified by the qadi of Beja, signed by an '*adl* (notary public), and sent to the authorities of Tunis.[4] And in March 1862 a certificate was issued by Lumbroso nominating 'Mohammed ben Tebib il Nafti della Provincia del Gerid' as 'Medico-Empirico' after he had passed an 'examination'[5] of an unspecified nature (see Fig. 6[b]).

Similar procedures were followed among the nomadic confederations such as the Drid in the north central region and the Farashish in the easternmost region. As late as 1880 applications from medical practitioners

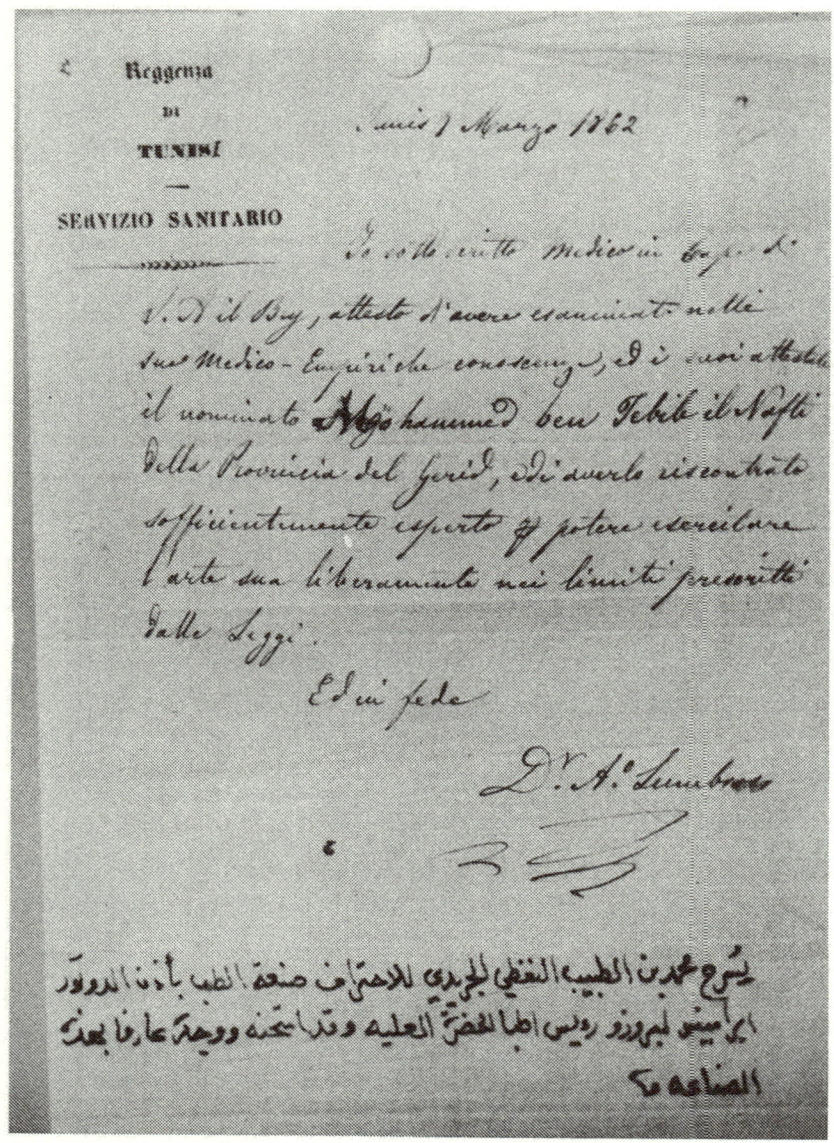

Fig. 6(b). Ijaza issued in 1862 to Muhammad b. Tabib al-Nefti by Abraham Lumbroso stating that the applicant can practice medicine within the limits prescribed by law

among the Drid and Farashish were carefully notarized locally and then submitted to the central authorities in Tunis.[6]

Muslim doctors licensed under the traditional system continued to serve in the maristan and later in the Sadiqi hospital. In 1861 Muhammad al-Kilani succeeded bu 'Asida, who had been amin al-atibba' since at least 1855, when he renewed al-Kilani's license. But he was amin in name only, retaining the position of head of the maristan but not licensor. Hamda Tabal al-Masakini followed al-Kilani, being appointed doctor of the maristan in 1871 and amin of circumcisors by beylical nomination (*amr*).[7] Hamda Tabal served as head of the maristan until his death in 1876. He was replaced by Qaddur b. Ahmad, the first European-trained Muslim doctor to practice in Tunisia.

Bin Ahmad, who was of Algerian origin, had studied at the French school of medicine at Algiers, where he had earned the degree of officer of health.[8] Upon completion of his studies, he immigrated to Tunis, possibly invited by Khayr al-Din. His family became well known and highly respected in the city of Tunis.

In 1876 he sent a note to Khayr al-Din, informing him of the death the day before of Si Hamda Tabal al-Masakini. In the letter he requested that he be appointed doctor of the maristan in his place.[9] The letter was a formality since he had been recruited for the post. Three years later Bin Ahmad became head of the new Mustashfa Sadiqi. Thus, the last official position in the medical establishment held by an empirical doctor passed to the hands of a European-trained Muslim, who had studied in a school in French-occupied Algeria. Bin Ahmad was succeeded by Bechir Dinguizli, who worked with a son of the former amin, Hamda b. Kilani, classed as *médecin toléré*, and with a second empiric, Muhammad Farah, classed as *attaché médecin adjoint* under the French occupation.[10]

Certain indigenous doctors were renowned for their skills. Hamda Tabal was widely respected and was mentioned in European accounts of colonial medical practice. The Kilani family had practiced medicine continuously since at least 1818, according to ijazas on record; it had provided an amin from 1861 to 1871 and finally a *médecin toléré*, a position created for non-European-trained doctors under the occupation. In losing the authority of the Muslim amin al-atibba', however, indigenous doctors were generally relegated to an inferior status often equated with that of quacks and charlatans. This situation contrasted with that of the early nineteenth century, when the opinion of the amin carried equal weight with that of the European doctor.

There were also numerous local Jewish medical practitioners, trained largely by experience. Gil Blass de Santillana and Elia Molco began as interpreters for licensed doctors and branched out on their own after

87

having learned some basic techniques and remedies.[11] A few, such as Vittorio Namia, were licensed by one of the European doctors.[12] Malaykhim Zaytun and David Attal were widely recognized; the latter went to France for retraining following the establishment of new regulations in the 1880s. The Attal family still provides medical specialists in modern Tunisia.

Expansion of European empirical medicine

The number of European empirics increased in the 1870s and 1880s, most practicing without a license. Most were charlatans with no medical training who came to seek their fortunes in the frontier-like conditions of post-1868 Tunisia. One, a French 'homeopath' named Burquet, set up practice in Tunis after failing as a photographer, shoe salesman, and circus director in Bone. He became Khaznadar's private doctor until the latter's death in 1878 and then served a brother of the bey.[13] On 1 December 1870, the arrival of an Italian homeopathic doctor was announced in *Ra'id al-tunisi*:

A new doctor has recently arrived [in Tunis]. He belongs to the school known by Westerners as 'homeopathy', which means to treat illnesses by something similar, or the use of medication that causes a disturbance in the human body similar to the illness which needs to be treated. This is contrary to the common school of the other group of doctors known as 'allopathy', which treats illness by contradiction, or the cooling of disease caused by fever and warming the temperature of disease caused by cold. ... The above is a brief summary of the announcement by Signor Cavalier Manidi, who has practiced plant chemistry and has spent time in Peru, Bolivia, and Argentina.

The similarity of homeopathic medicine to local Arabic medical ideas is striking. Galenic medical concepts, shared by Europeans and Muslims until the nineteenth century, are explicit in the definition of allopathic medicine. By 1870, however, such theories were considered outmoded by most medical experts in Europe.

Like other medical fashions emanating from Europe, patent medicines were brought to Tunisia by traveling salesman–doctors. One remedy advertised in the Arabic newspaper was good for the liver and stomach, for counteracting yellow fever, and for strengthening weak bodies. It was available at an Italian pharmacy in Tunis. Foreigners from non-European regions apparently encountered difficulty in attracting clients. In the early 1860s a Turkish doctor submitted a petition to the government asking for funds to send himself and his family back to Istanbul since there was no work for him in Tunis.[14]

This expansion of empirical medicine was contested by the bey's personal physician at the time, Giacomo Castelnuovo. Like Lumbroso, he was of Livornese–Jewish parentage and from a family well established in Tunisia. In addition to pursuing his medical career Castelnuovo founded a bank in Florence and in 1868 negotiated a commercial treaty between Italy and Tunis. He represented Sadiq Bey in negotiations that led to the establishment of the International Financial Commission in 1869. For his efforts he was ennobled by Victor Emmanuel II and awarded mining concessions in Tunisia by Sadiq Bey. A French merchant complained that the backing of Castelnuovo and his compatriots at court enabled the Livornese merchants to gain preference over French merchants by their ability to 'play on many tables at the same time'.[15] Castelnuovo was intensely involved in business affairs in Tunisia. Perhaps as a representative of European civilization, he saw himself as an agent of progress.

In 1877 Castelnuovo published a letter addressed to Khayr al-Din in the *Journal officiel tunisien*. In his letter he noted that the number of indigenous and European empirics and pharmacists had multiplied since his arrival in Tunisia thirty-three years earlier. At that time there were only two pharmacies, one run by a French chemist and the other by an empiric under the direction of an Italian.

But now with the expansion of medicine and an enlightened prime minister, he urged the government to enact a law to control the practice of medicine and pharmacy in the country he had come to regard as a second home. He noted that 'the modern bibliography of hygiene numbered 679 volumes and that no government bordering on Europe was without laws regulating medicine and pharmacy nor lacked a code for a sanitary administration'. Wherever, he said, progress had begun to dissipate the shadows of ignorance and superstition, the governments had established a set of rules specifically to assure and to protect the public health, which was the foundation of the state.[16]

Castelnuovo was advocating legitimization of the European biomedical tradition as the sole medical system in Tunisia. But by the mid-1870s there were only about twenty European doctors practicing in Tunisia, nearly all of whom were Italian, for a population of 1.5 million.[17] At the time Castelnuovo wrote his letter, a team of Italian experts was ostentatiously exploring the country, preparing a report on its resources and developmental prospects. Castelnuovo himself was in Tunisia to supervise development of the Jabal Rasas lead mine, a concession he had obtained for his participation in the 1868 commercial negotiations, and of the tuna fishing industry, in which he had invested 50,000 piasters.[18] In effect, he considered medical reform a preliminary phase of economic colonization. Tunisia was expected to become a modern state under Italian tutelage.

Muslim medical reforms

Tunisian reformers such as the Mamluk prime minister Khayr al-Din al-Tunisi were acutely aware of the danger posed by the European ascendancy. They had lived through the difficulties caused by the 1867–8 epidemics and were aware of European medical advances. In his program for reform, *The Surest Path*, Khayr al-Din cited numerous achievements by European medical researchers.[19] Though the causes of the epidemic diseases were still unknown in the 1870s, the connection between disease and sanitation had been well established. Khayr al-Din, in Castelnuovo's words, was 'enlightened' though not working toward the same goals. Khayr al-Din was anxious to enact measures that would strengthen his state, the better to resist further encroachment by foreign interests. Though he was unable to put through a law regulating the practice of medicine prior to his dismissal in 1877, he was working toward reorganization of urban sanitation procedures and expansion of the maristan.

On 2 July 1872 a Sanitation Service for the city of Tunis had been officially announced through Khayr al-Din's efforts. A beylical decree placed the *ad hoc* Sanitary Police, which had been formed by the European communities in the 1860s, under Tunisian administration. The Muslim president of the Municipal Council, al-'Arbi Zarruq, presided over the Sanitary Service Committee (*majlis al-nazafa*), which was composed of consular representatives and shaykhs of the quarters. The Municipal Council imposed a new property tax to support the activities of the Sanitation Service. But the Italians and Maltese who made up the majority of the foreign communities refused to pay the tax and after further negotiations their consuls forced an agreement whereby the moneys were collected. The council then formed a Municipal Sanitary Police Corps to enforce these measures along with other urban ordinances. Under the auspices of the committee, major streets were paved and certain public buildings were repaired.[20] But the open-air drains remained in use and in winter the lower streets of the city became mires of mud and refuse as usual. The Sanitary Council continued to complain that the city was a foyer of infection and that typhus, which appeared again in 1874, would transmute into bubonic plague in the poisoned soil.[21]

Khayr al-Din and Bayram al-Khamis, now rector of the Great Mosque and wakil of waqf funds, then made plans for the expansion of the maristan, which was still functioning as it had since 1662. It was far too small for a city of about 100,000 inhabitants. But the waqf funds for the maristan were exhausted after the trials of the 1860s, and in the early 1870s the salaries of the staff had been reduced.[22] In 1872 an additional tax was thus imposed to collect revenues for the projected hospital, which was clearly a necessity if the Muslim majority was to have services comparable to those of the European communities.

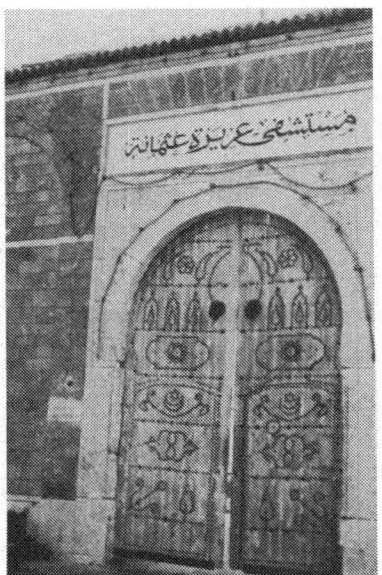 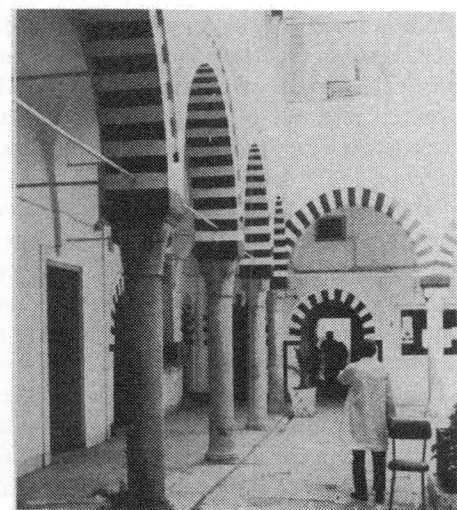

Fig. 7. Sadiqi hospital. (a) exterior; (b) interior

After numerous delays the new hospital was finally opened in 1879, an event celebrated with great fanfare. The bey officially opened the hospital, with dignitaries of the European communities and representatives from the Muslim quarters attending. Newspapers carried the new waqf provisions and descriptions of the establishment. The Mustashfa Sadiqi was named after the reigning bey, but, like the old maristan, it was popularly referred to as Mustashfa 'Aziza 'Uthmana after the seventeenth-century benefactress. It was housed in a refurbished Janissary barracks located near the citadel of the Kasbah, the site of the government. It was much larger than the older hospice, with a hundred beds and special rooms for the mentally ill, the sick sent from prisons, and the indigent sick. Eighteen beds were reserved for women. The hospital had a pharmacy, a room for operations, a hammam, garden, and mosque. The waqfs, which were supplemented by the tax, amounted to 150,000 piasters annually.[23]

Medicine and colonial domination

In the 1870s, Tunisian reformers were hastily trying to revise and strengthen indigenous political, military, educational, and medical institutions to withstand deepening European domination. Meanwhile Britain, France, and Germany were working out compromises that would allow further colonial ventures. In 1881 a French cavalry detachment sent from Algeria to quell a border disturbance continued until it reached Tunis, where it was joined by an expedition that had landed in Bizerte. To quieten local and international protests the initial occupation was said to be temporary, lasting until the bey could guarantee the security of his borders and the protection of the 700 French residents in Tunis. The protectorate was officially arranged in 1883, but French intentions had been clear since invasion was first planned during the dismal years of 1867–8.

Following the occupation the consular Sanitary Council continued to meet, concerning itself with repairing lazarets, quarantining pilgrims returning from Mecca, disinfecting the waters of Zaghouan, and cleaning the streets of the city. Complaints had been filed against the Jewish empiric Nomo, who was port doctor at La Goulette after They's departure, and in 1880 the ubiquitous Castelnuovo was elected doctor of sanitation at the port. Epidemics remained a major concern in the 1880s; plague was announced in Baghdad in 1881 and cholera broke out in Mecca in 1882 during the month of pilgrimage. The disease spread through parts of the Middle East and Europe and was soon in Marseilles and Toulon.[24]

In September 1884 the major of Tunis, Muhammad al-Umbaza, sent an order to the Medical Corps concerning procedures for the disinfection and purification of the city. Books of white and tinted paper were issued for daily reporting of cases of cholera.[25] The city braced itself for the onslaught but months passed without a case. When the disease struck Malta, the occupying government decided to take over the functions of the now fifty-year-old Sanitary Council.

In a decree of 20 February 1885 Muhammad al-'Aziz bu 'Attur, the prime minister, in consultation with Paul Cambon, the resident-minister, promulgated a law instituting a Maritime Sanitary Police which began with this preamble: 'The administration of sanitation of the Regency, the utility of which was recognized during the epidemic of cholera which had reached a part of Europe, is the object of our gratitude. The rapid development of commerce and frequent communications with countries situated to the north of the Mediterranean necessitates the organization of a service installed and directed by a permanent chief. On the other hand, it appears useful to consult the interested parties on sanitary questions so we have, with the support of the French government, issued this decree.'[26]

In 113 articles provisions for quarantining and inspection of Tunisia's three lazarets were put forth. Cholera, yellow fever, and plague were to be quarantined and typhus and smallpox were not. The new Sanitary Council was to be composed of the administrators, scientists, and merchants who would be most capable of enlightened judgment in questions concerning public health. The government appointed two consuls, two members of the Municipal Council, two members from the Chamber of Commerce, and two doctors. The first four nominated were administrators Yusuf Ja'it and Ahmad al-Hawan and doctors Deloulme and Spezzafumo. Dr Gariel became director of health, and Pelluet and Ornano were appointed police commissioners at the ports of La Goulette and Bizerte; positions of coercion were to be held by Europeans.[27]

Official attitudes toward indigenous practitioners now reflected the new colonial relationship. In 1884 T. Poncet, director of the health service of the Division of Occupation, addressed a letter to M. Bompard, secretary general of the Tunisian government, in which he recommended a study entitled *On the Criminality of the Arabs*. The study was prepared at the Faculty of Medicine at Lyon under the direction of one of his friends, Prof. La Cassagne. It contained 'very curious documents relative to the legal Arab medicine' which he thought should enlighten certain points of justice in difficult cases concerning local medical practices.[28]

Indigenous and European empirical medicine was legally curtailed by the decree of 15 June 1888, which regulated medicine, surgery, and obstetrics. It declared that all persons who had practiced medicine for five years or less in Tunisia had to prove that they had completed at least three years of medical school. Each additional year was equivalent to a year of practice. Indigenous practitioners under sixty years of age who had practiced for at least twenty years were allowed to continue if they had an ijaza from the bey. Indigenous doctors who practiced in towns where there were no licensed doctors were allowed to continue without an ijaza, but could not perform surgery.[29]

The days when European doctors sought to stay on good terms with the amin al-atibba' to avoid trouble were gone. Now, indigenous doctors such as Hamda b. Kilani, son of the former amin, were classed as *médecins tolérés*. Members of the new medical elite were licensed only in Europe. Italian doctors continued to predominate until the early twentieth century, when there were about twenty French doctors. By 1928 there were only ten French-trained Tunisian doctors in Tunisia. The majority of the licensed French, Italian, and Tunisian doctors practiced in Tunis.[30]

The Muslim hospital, Mustashfa Sadiqi, did not become the modern equivalent of the French hospital. Its funds proved inadequate, and although the new location was more spacious and better ventilated and the mats replaced with mattresses, the food and pharmacy were scarcely improved over those of the maristan, and the hospital remained the last resort of the sick.

In 1892, when F. Lovy, a new doctor to the bey, arrived in Tunis, there were only thirty-eight patients, most tubercular, paralytic, or blind. In the twenty-five years since the head of the hospital, Qaddur b. Ahmad, had received his training, anesthetics and other medical advances had been introduced. With use of the new techniques, the clientele increased.[31] The first French-trained Tunisian doctor, Bechir Dinguizli, was to begin his practice at the hospital in 1894. The waqf funds were supplemented with additional funds at the turn of the century and the hospital has since been enlarged. Today it is a major regional hospital, but popularly considered inferior to the French hospitals. Two smaller waqf-supported hospices at Sfax and Sousse remained in use into the early twentieth century. The takiyas, founded in 1775 by 'Ali Bey, were expanded in 1919 and 1922 with waqf funds.[32]

In 1880 Sadiq Bey had granted another barracks in the central city to Cardinal Lavigerie for use as a European hospital. It replaced the small hospital founded by Abbé Bourgade in 1841 near the Great Mosque. The hospital had only eight beds and was staffed by volunteer doctors and the Sisters of Saint Joseph. The new, larger establishment was named Hôpital Saint Louis and in 1897 became the Hôpital Civil Français. It was recently moved outside the city and renamed Hôpital Charles Nicolle, after Nicolle's discovery at Sadiqi hospital of the role of lice in transmitting typhus. A Jewish hospital was founded in 1894 to serve the large indigenous community hitherto served by the Italian or Sadiqi hospitals.[33] It was considered of intermediate quality, better than the Muslim hospital, but worse than the French hospital, thus reflecting the new colonial hierarchy.

With perhaps one doctor per 50,000 inhabitants at the turn of the century, most of the population had recourse only to empirical medicine. Indigenous pharmacists continued to give consultations in the herb *suqs* (markets) of Tunis and other market centers, barbers bled clients who were ailing, and bonesetters repaired fractures. Home remedies such as honey, olive oil, henna, lemon juice, and rose water remained in use. And zawiyas provided a medical context that existed nearly outside French control.

The Sufi zawiyas became an important source of social welfare as the ruling elite turned to Western medicine and legislated against the empirical practitioners, because this alternative system could treat illnesses beyond the purview of Western medicine. Certain zawiyas continued to perform exorcisms for their clients, and there were many stories of successes where Western medicine had failed. The occupying government viewed the zawiyas as fonts of resistance and tried to suppress the more active for their 'nonorthodoxy'. In 1911 pilgrimages to a shrine outside Tunis were forbidden during a smallpox epidemic, officially for fear of disease communication. But after the cessation of the outbreak the interdiction was maintained. The policy was defended on the basis that the ceremonies encouraged pro-Muslim, anti-French sentiments and that donations collected would be used to oppose the government's political direction.[34]

The government hoped that French medicine would be an effective substitute for the missionary work which failed to gain many religious or cultural converts in Muslim North Africa. A French doctor concluded his 1855 study of Arab medicine in Algeria with a discussion of the potential civilizing role of European medicine from a political, humanitarian, and scientific point of view. He says France had not only a military conquest but also a moral conquest to undertake: 'There are prejudices to modify, errors to correct, ignorance to dissipate, misery and apathy to destroy...new needs to create....' He asks if it is not 'good politics to oppose the pretended "omni-science" of the marabouts with the influence – not religious, but positive and practical – of men capable and strong in their knowledge?' French medicine can bring 'above all in case of epidemics, energetic help which will impress the unbelievers and empirics by rapidly obtained results...'.[35]

European medicine became an integral part of the French *mission civilisatrice* as it had earlier been a part of foreign policy, facilitating political influence and economic expansion. The *Revue tunisienne* (1905) observed that 'the doctor is the true conqueror, the peaceful conqueror.... It follows that if we wish to penetrate their hearts, to win the confidence of the Muslims, it is in multiplying the services of medical assistance that we will arrive at it most surely.' A 1904 essay on French medical assistance in Tunisia claimed that 'nothing serves better our influence than the medical institutions and with the aid of doctors, one does a good work for humanity which is also good for France; it is double profit'.[36]

The nineteenth-century epidemics themselves were not only a motivation for public health reforms but also, for colonial historians, a proof of the failure of Islamic rule. Propagandists now found French rule to be legitimate and necessary if only for medical reasons. In 1912 a French medical journal expounded this new version of history:

North Africa, which had been very healthy under the Roman occupation, saw its sanitary conditions change from day to day during the long Arab–Turkish nightmare. We have witnessed continual wars, and bloody revolutions, and we have seen the most formidable calamities follow one another during the long centuries. In the middle of such miseries, epidemics have struck fatally. They found a wondrous terrain among these poor beings, emaciated by hunger, poorly clothed, living in conditions of lamentable hygiene.

When one thinks of ways so primitive that our consuls themselves had to try to check the plagues, when one thinks also of the habitual indifference of Muslims which results totally from fatalism, one understands why contagious diseases caused such ravages during the long centuries.[37]

By the beginning of the twentieth century two myths had become cornerstones of colonial history: the myth of Muslim fatalism and the myth of European medicine coming to the rescue. Actually, in Tunisia the beys and Muslim reformers had tried to follow those procedures they thought most apt to succeed in disease defense, regardless of their cultural or national origin. The Tunisian authorities hoped to learn from European medical expertise how better to deal with epidemics, the consequences of which were, ironically, exacerbated by the European impact. They did not intend to lose their power to foreign occupation as part of Europeanization. Following the occupation, however, the French government was able to legislate medical reform on its own terms and to propagate its own ideology of the role of medicine in the colonial process.

Conclusion

Social historians have seized upon epidemics and their effects on people's lives as fundamental causes or 'motors of human history' and as unique sources of historical insight. In the case of Tunisia from 1780 to 1900, epidemics were indeed of major significance, being barometers of social change, catalysts of medical reform, and even justification for political power. But contrary to the analyses of many contemporary observers and modern historians, the epidemics did not cause the economic destabilization that characterized the history of nineteenth-century Tunisia.

Mortality and history

Following the severe plague of 1785–6, the Tunisian economy apparently fared well, and there was no political instability that can be associated with the high mortality caused by the disease. The economic recession that followed the 1818–20 plague resulted from complex international commercial and political developments that reversed Tunisia's trade advantages. In the 1830s and 1840s, a succession of unequal trade treaties imposed by militarily superior European powers led the beys to instigate multifaceted reforms that stressed expansion of their own armed forces. Increased taxes to support the reforms and to redress public (governmental) loss of commercial revenue further distorted the indigenous economy. The agricultural recession that accompanied the 1849–50 cholera epidemic was largely a consequence of overtaxation and lack of investment capital. Immediately following the 1856 epidemic, agriculture prospered due to regularized taxation and favorable weather. In 1867–8, the cholera and typhus epidemics precipitated bankruptcy and foreign takeover of Tunisian finances. But the underlying causes of bankruptcy were the internationally generated economic crises, popular revolt, its suppression, and the famine of 1865–6. Epidemics in nineteenth-century Tunisia played a role that was significant but not crucial in historical causation.

Epidemics and social change

If epidemics are not necessarily motors of history, are they nevertheless mirrors of history? Social responses to the series of epidemic diseases indicate a fundamental shift in public confidence in persons considered responsible in time of crisis. During the plague epidemics of 1784–5, the government consulted the 'ulama' on legal questions related to the European practice of quarantining, and the 'ulama' took the side of public opinion in opposition to the bey's orders. Likewise in the 1818–20 epidemic, the 'ulama' issued statements that were carefully studied regarding the imposition of the sanitary cordon around the city. Even in the 1849–50 cholera epidemic, when Ahmad Bey enforced strict quarantines and other public health measures, the Hanafi qadi ordered forty men named Muhammad, all descended from the Prophet, to recite an invocation to curtail the disease. By the 1860s, the 'ulama' were no longer consulted, and the European-run quarantine service had become an institution within the Tunisian government. After the 1860s epidemics, Tunisian reformers tried to institute European-style medical and public health reforms with the clear intention of replacing the old medical system. Traditional forms of Islamic science and medicine were now less valid, and new ideas were personified by Europeans themselves. At the beginning of the nineteenth century, the 'ulama' were the ultimate guardians of scientific knowledge and of received wisdom. By the end of the century, Europeans were the undisputed guardians of science and technology.

The rising position of European doctors relative to Muslim doctors reflected the shift to dependency on European political, economic, and scientific authority. In the eighteenth century, both Muslim and European doctors were given official recognition as head of the doctors' order and the maristan and as physician to the bey respectively. By 1861, Muslim doctors had to be licensed by the bey's European physician, and in 1876, a European-trained Muslim doctor assumed the directorship of the maristan. Following the establishment of the colonial government, Europeans themselves took over the direct management of institutions of medicine and public health.

The choice of medical personnel was long influenced by the position of European nations at court. In the eighteenth century, many court doctors were French. By the mid-nineteenth century, with the rise of Italian commerce, most were Italian. Following the occupation of 1881, the issue was settled: the medical system not only was reformed along Western lines but was run by and largely for the French colonial elite.

By the end of the nineteenth century, the ancient Arabic medical structure had vanished with scarcely a trace.

Epidemics and medical reform

Equally important for the social historian is the most direct consequence of epidemic disease: the medical response. Many of the medical innovations of the eighteenth and nineteenth centuries resulted from the threat of epidemics that destroyed troops and workers. Medical change is, however, caused only in part by demonstrable efficacy: political and economic interests and cultural assumptions all influence medical options. In Tunisia, the epidemics stimulated medical reform, and today they reveal for the historian the dynamics of medical change shaped by the historical context of the times. The unequal power conflict that engulfed the Mediterranean dictated the actual formation of medical structures.

From the eighteenth century, the elite's choice of European physicians was, for example, influenced not only by the unrealized hope that they could cure endemic and epidemic disease but by the expectation that they could provide special diplomatic services. Doctors such as Lumbroso and Castelnuovo played four roles at once: disinterested medical consultant, employee and confidant of the bey, government agent, and entrepreneur with privileged ties to court. The facilitation of trade was in fact a central interest of court doctors and their European consuls. In time of epidemic, beys, doctors, and consuls generally supported the imposition of quarantine procedures. Quarantines, however, not only prevented contact with disease but also impeded commerce and travel, and this created suspicion and resentment. When, in 1835, the bey's authority to impose quarantines passed into the hands of the European consuls, a fundamental shift in power relationships had taken place reflecting new commercial realities and a need to mediate rival interests among the now dominant European powers. The bey had no choice but to endorse this loss of power and to cooperate with the consular representatives on the Sanitary Council. The bey's interests lay in the continuity of the established order, even if the new base of political legitimacy was accommodation with the European powers. European economic colonization was a threat in the years following the Napoleonic Wars, and the Muslim elite decided that European-style modernization would help resist further exploitation and strengthen their own power.

Following the epidemics of the 1860s and the establishment of European financial control, Tunisian reformers made public health reform a central aspect of their program. The disastrous epidemics and perhaps the knowledge that European capital cities were generally more prosperous and had public health programs convinced reformers that new sanitary laws and provisions like those enacted by European municipal governments were necessary. Furthermore, during the epidemics, the European communities had become nearly autonomous and self-governing in matters of public health maintenance, and the reformers wished to forestall this tendency by bringing all aspects of government back under Tunisian supervision.

The medical and public health theories and practices (contagion, miasma, subsidized medicine, public sanitation laws) were not foreign. Both Arabic and European medical remedies *c.* 1800 centered on herbal remedies and phlebotomy. In Tunisia, public health reforms first consisted of improving older institutions and increasing waqf funding. Tunisia was, however, subject to the same medical fashions as Europe: during the course of the century, homeopathy came and went, patent medicines advertised by itinerant salesmen came into temporary vogue, European medical empirics flourished despite their lack of formal medical training. During the epidemics, Muslim doctors began to incorporate remedies like quinine and mercury from European doctors. Europeans in turn tried local treatments like scarification for treating cholera victims. With the shift in confidence from Arabic to European medicine, the Muslim political elite intended merely to learn from their mentors while retaining political control. But they too were overthrown in the tide of Europeanization.

In 1888, new laws curtailing the practice of indigenous medicine placed medical change in a different light. There was now a dichotomy along ethnic lines: legal, European medicine, supported by the French colonial government; and semilegal, Arabic medicine, utilized by most of the populace. At the time there were no European-trained Tunisian doctors and perhaps twenty European doctors, nearly all residing in Tunis. European medicine had become a first-class system associated with the wealthy ruling elite. Arabic medicine had become a second-class system patronized mostly by those outside the privileged sector.

Medicine and political legitimacy

In the colonial era, the link between scientific knowledge and power was never in doubt. All governments need to justify themselves, and the French government stressed the necessity for political change through the damage wrought by the epidemics. Colonial propagandists made the medical transition a part of imperialist ideology: Tunisians, like other Muslims, because of religion and culture, were said to be passive or fatalistic in the face of epidemic disease and so stood to gain from guidance by a more enlightened civilization. The medical efforts of the eighteenth- and nineteenth-century beys and Muslim reformers were quietly forgotten.

It was, nevertheless, the Muslim leadership who effected the initial stages of the reform process. Why was there so little protest against this by the indigenous medical doctors? The amin al-atibba' was dependent upon the bey's nomination so when the bey nominated his European physician to the role, there was no basis for appeal. Furthermore, because of the paucity of European-trained doctors, indigenous Muslim doctors lost their legal status but not their clientele.

By 1900, Europeans dominated the medical establishment. Arabic medical practitioners were officially discredited. The transition to European medicine, like the economic reversal, was a result more of the process of colonization than of the struggle with epidemic disease. During the economic and political rivalries of the late eighteenth and early nineteenth centuries, medicine had proven to be both a function of power and a tool in the struggle for power.

Waqf (hubus) document for the maristan of Tunis[1]

Praise be to God, in whose hands is weakness and strength, and the creation of sickness and medicine, who created bodies for atonement of sin, who brings recompense and averts disaster, who knows what is clear and what is hidden, and what is in all hearts. Peace be upon his noble Prophet, his great healer, Muhammad, especially God's beloved, but universal in his mission of call, root of remedy, pole of the circle of his wisdom, source of cure, free of whim in the eloquence of his word, as stated in Sura 'al-Najma idha hawa'. Peace be upon his pure family and on his venerable companions, the stars of guidance and the base of piety.

When the chain of possibilities was linked to the presence of God, the Blessed and Almighty, thus order in every kingdom was organized by the presence of an *amir* [ruler] or khalifa as the base of power and security against the mishaps of time; thus God granted such an amir to the land of Tunis and Africa; a man from the select, shadow of justice who created for the multitudes kind deeds which he brought forth into being. He prevented by his policy the ruses of those of injustice and tyranny; he cleared the roads of fear and enmity with the awe of his policies, until men and boys, and women and girls, traveled upon them. How often he hit those who hit him with the accurate arrow of his bow. And he hit the target in the jugular vein. How much those who returned to him profited by his relation and from his vast bounty. He is the faithful lord, the clearest flag, the famous, the elite of the amirs of the past; gem of the dynasties of the *basha*s [pashas] of the past, organizer of the famous Tunisian army and master of the flying flag. One who has authority and is direct in word and deed, [he is] Sayyid Abu 'Abd Allah Muhammad Basha, may God help him and protect his subjects; make long for the Muslims the security by making last his leadership. May his name be praised, with concern for his great policies and sound leadership, he who seeks to draw near [to God] by means of sacrifice, by providing charity for the needy and for those in want, with ample, continous alms, and everlasting, virtuous hubus. His lofty zeal is devoted to it. His noble view was directed toward it and by attention to the condition of the poor, and mercy for the predicament of the weak and the sick, he created a maristan to repair to and to provide medicine and food and what is needed by them.

He established as its properties the following:

1. The south funduq opening near the Qabaqabiyyin and the school of 'Azzafin

within Tunis, bordered on the south where the open land is, and east by the property of Da'isi, and north by the property of the *mu'adhdhin* [muezzin] al-Hajj Muhammad al-Qassir and others, and west by the road with its rights and uses. All the revenues from the following:

2. The six shops included in the limits above.
3. The oven now used for baking [in this area].
4. The kiln...[further information omitted from the published document].
5. The north funduq....
6. The two shops opening from the above-mentioned funduq....
7. The north storehouses....
8. The east kiln....
9. The east shop....
10. The south kiln....
11. The south funduq....
12. The two east shops....
13. The funduq of the two doors....
14. The funduq west of the gate....
15. The hammam west of the newly built gate being in the city of Le Kef.
16. The five shops adjoining it....
17. The water drawn from the spring known as the spring of Sidi Salem....
18. The water coming from the above-mentioned hammam....
19. The hammam west of the open space in the city of Zaghouan....
20. The four pipes of water coming from the above-mentioned city....
21. The south oven used for baking bread in the city of Le Kef....
22. The west mill used for milling food in Le Kef....
23. The east hammam in the square of Bizerte....
24. The kiln and house adjoining it outside the city of Beja....
25. The west funduq in Beja....
26. Half of the house north of the gate located in the Jewish quarter, inside Bab Suwayqa in Tunis, the protected....

It is confirmed now like this in the presence of two *shahid*s [witnesses], by al-Sayyid, the great and noble, our lord Abu 'Abd Allah Muhammad Basha, master of the throne of the city of Tunis, who now places his seal here. He is the owner of all the yields delineated above, may his loftiness be increased. Son of the deceased amir, the great, who has passed to the mercy of God, [is] our lord, Abu al-Za'far Murad Basha, may God sanctify his soul and let him dwell in the highest heaven. He testifies that he has established a hubus and waqf of all the revenues delineated above with all their rights and benefits, their yield, and what is attached to them as outlined below in detail:

The aforesaid funduq is made into a maristan as a place to shelter the sick and the wounded from sea expeditions or mahallas or *ghazwa*s [raids] for the sake of God, and for the poor of those who have no money and no one to take care of them and no shelter in the city of Tunis; [it is to be] a place where the sick of those mentioned above can find care; where they can stay until completely cured. When one of the sick people is cured of his illness, and the doctor announces news of his cure, the supervisor of the maristan mentioned above will dismiss him. There is to be no distinction among the sick and wounded, be they Arab, non-Arab [a'jami], Turkish, or any other. The remainder of the yield mentioned above is entirely to be spent as is said and outlined below:

For what is necessary of food and medicine appropriate to the condition of each and for the servants to care for them night and day until the end, and likewise what they need of bedding and covers, straw matting, mattresses, safsaris, and wool covers for winter and linen for summer. Those of the ill whom God destines to die in the maristan will be provided with what is needed of shrouds, burial and interment. He [the bey], may God preserve him, has appointed an expert doctor to treat them. He has for this what he needs of potions, herbs, oils, ointments, bandages, and a room in the maristan in which to sit, and eight nasris and four loaves of bread each day. Also, a man is provided for them as overseer of expenses and for him are four nasris and two loaves of bread each day; a cook to cook for them their food, meat and other things, for him are five nasris and two loaves of bread each day; the man who stays in the maristan night and day as bawwab to lock the doors, sweep the courtyard and open space, to draw water for drinking and washing, and to wash the clothing of the sick and other than that as is needed for them earns eight nasris and four loaves of bread each day. The bread loaves are to be worth a nasri in good times and bad.

[The bey] has made as hubus all the revenues mentioned above and has made them waqf for those specified, with all their rights and benefits according to sacred law, as perpetual waqf forever, which cannot be sold nor given away until God inherits the earth, and he is the best of inheritors. There is to be no change in its condition, nor organization until God inherits it, continuing its sources, preserving its conditions. He who changes it after what he has heard has sinned against those who established it. God is all-hearing and all-knowing. He rewards those who give alms and money given in alms is not lost.

All this comes after funds have been taken out of the revenues for building and repair so that it remains standing on its foundation benefiting from it. [The bey] has given supervision of [the hubus fund] to his two sons, Murad Bey, *sahib al-mahalla* [commander of the mahalla], and Sayyid Abu 'Abd Allah Muhammad Bey, master of the *sanjaq* [district] of the city of Kairouan, Sousse, Monastir, Sfax, and the two cities of the Sahel. Then to the oldest and the next oldest, and to the most pious of their brothers, then to their children and their children's children, and their issue and the issue of their issue whom they beget and the expansion of their branches in Islam. The people of lower class are not before people of higher class in supervision even if they are older. May God preserve the present supervisor of the maristan, the worthy Musa Khamira al-Andalusi, who is given responsibility in this and possession of all the yields as said, and who is present and accepts it completely. He transfers it in reward to the other world. It is testified by their testimony in legal condition as waqf on the above-mentioned establishment as stated, in the middle of Rabi' al-Awal, made noble by [the Prophet's] birth, 1073 [29 October 1662] with the knowledge of the supervisor, and the complete knowledge of Sayyid Muhammad Basha, in the witness of the two just jurists, the shaykhs Abu 'Abd Allah Muhammad al-Mahrazi and the mufti, 'Abd Allah Naji. This is an exact copy of that; if one compares this with the original document, he will see that they are exact copies. This is testified to here in the beginning of Dhu al-Hijja 1100 [September 1689]. Signatures of two witnesses follow.

Appendix B

Letter from Husayn Bey to de Lesseps on reasons for the quarantine

From the slave of god...the living king, our lord, Husayn Basha Bey, master of the kingdom of Tunis...to our ally, Cavalier Mathieu de Lesseps, consul general of France in Tunis:

Your letter reached us on 2 Rabi' Ithani 1244 [12 December 1828]. In it you referred to a letter from your country concerning the ten days' quarantine which we ordered for all merchant ships coming to our country to save the people from outbreaks of disease. Your request was to remove the quarantine from merchant ships coming from your Mediterranean ports. We have considered your request and the answer is that we have ordered the ten days to protect the people. God Almighty gave us the duty to take care of their welfare and to protect them from contagious diseases.

It came to us from many authoritative sources that plague, yellow fever, and other diseases are spreading. Yellow fever is severe in Gibraltar and elsewhere. We know that merchant ships have contact with other ships at sea and in port so we ordered these ten days to protect the land and the people. As for the corsair ships with their long stays at sea, we ordered any corsair ship to return to its port of origin for twenty days and to carry a patent in its language in the hand of its captain, who must prove the ship had no contact with another at sea and visited no other port. If the captain can prove it we will accept it. We put this order on all types of ships coming to our country. Orders cannot be done for some and not others. If we accept your request, others would demand it and enforcing the order would become very difficult. The result would be corruption coming to our country....

[Postscript]

France, with its ancient friendship with us, understands we did not order the quarantine to hinder commerce. We made the order not knowing if it will work, but it might, so it is not possible for us not to do it....

Epidemics and population trends

Contemporary observers frequently offered the recurring epidemics of the nineteenth century as an explanation for Tunisia's increasing weakness. Close analysis suggests that the sharp demographic decline cited by contemporaries and later by historians did not in fact take place. Mortality rates, however, confirm the importance of the epidemics as major historical events that, because of the context of the times, did lead to new forms of medicine and public health.

Population size

Contemporary estimates of the population of Tunisia during the nineteenth century range from 800,000 (Pellissier de Reynaud in 1853) to 5,000,000 (Duveyier in 1881); most fall within a range of one to two million.[1] Verification of such estimates is hazardous; the lack of systematic method in collecting the figures tends to disqualify them. Most were at best obtained after a quick journey on horseback through rural regions and quick tours through towns where dwellings were haphazardly counted. The depopulation that witnesses ascribed to epidemic crises can be understood in part as a result of temporary migrations. At times, the migrations were to the cities in search of famine relief from food distribution centers. Settled and seminomadic groups often sought escape from increasingly heavy taxation, government repression, or bad living conditions by migrating toward Libya or Algeria. In 1853 Pellissier de Reynaud observed that 'settled peoples had shown a great tendency to emigrate toward the tribes and their relative autonomy.... If the government does not find a remedy for this, it will find itself in a very embarrassing situation.'[2] Populations moved but they did not disappear. Most returned to their homes after a few months when conditions had stabilized.

Most historians have accepted Jean Ganiage's population estimates: 1.1 million total population in 1860 and 80,000 in Tunis, figures based on extrapolation from the 1856 and 1860 tax censuses.[3] While recent demographic analyses indicate that the city size estimate is too low, projection back in time from the 1921 census tends to corroborate the total population estimate. As Tunisian demographer Mahmud Seklani has observed, population growth rates were in all probability 0.0 percent from 1860 to 1865 and 0.8 to 1.2 percent from 1875 to 1922. These rates reflect the series of political, economic, and epidemiological crises that prevented substantial population increase.[4]

Applying standard demographic formulas for projection back in time and using the uncorrected 1921 census figure of 1,874,981 (Muslim population), we find that the probable population size in 1875 was between 1,016,000 (assuming a high birth rate) and 1,247,000 (assuming a low birth rate).[5] Capital city population estimates by contemporary observers were generally more accurate simply because the traveler or government official remained there longer. Moreover, certain contemporaries were in an excellent position to estimate the population accurately. Lumbroso placed the total population of Tunis at 150,000 to 200,000 in 1850.[6] In a consular report of 8 July 1867, P. M. S. Werry, a British consular official and careful observer, reported that the city had 150,000 inhabitants.[7] Other sources vary from 80,000 to 150,000 including residents of all religions.[8] Recent demographic analyses have tended to support the higher population estimates. In his 1974 study André Raymond accepted a figure of 100,000 to 150,000 for Tunis from 1830 to 1881, based on his correlations of the number of hammams per person in Tunis with the ratio in other Islamic–Mediterranean cities.[9] In his 1971 study, André Lézine estimated the population of Tunis in 1896 at 160,000 from the number of buildings and from historical accounts.[10] An early but competent demographic study undertaken in 1898 counted 100,000 Muslim, 30,000 Jewish, and 29,000 European inhabitants.[11] A preliminary 1906 census counted a total population of 204,500 in Tunis, of whom 61,000 were European.[12] The protectorate government, established in 1881, may have overcounted the European population and undercounted the Muslim population.

Paul Sebag, noted historian of Tunisia, estimates that during the eighteenth century the population increased to about 2 to 2.5 million, but as a result of the 1784–5 and 1818–20 plague epidemics, it dropped to under 1.5 million.[13] From the contemporary accounts, such figures appear reasonable.

Population trends

According to the eighteenth-century chronicler Hamuda Ibn 'Abd al-'Aziz, formerly vacant lands around Tunis were turned into city suburbs and the government authorized the construction of new markets and roads. Population growth was visible to all, not only in the cities, but also in the countryside, where the amount of land under cultivation expanded. Contemporaries attributed the population increase to an unprecedented reprieve from plague epidemic between 1705 and 1784.[14] In his 1971 study, however, Lézine found the population increase to be a continuation of a five-hundred-year trend not greatly affected by epidemics.[15]

The population increase was apparently curbed by the severe plagues of 1784–5 and 1818–20. A letter from the French consul in Tunis announced that a third of the inhabitants of Tunisia had died in the earlier epidemic.[16] The vice-consul of Holland, Nyssen, who was also in Tunis during the epidemic, reported to Vicheret that 300,000 had perished in Tunis and a million in Tunisia.[17] This is more than the total population of the capital city and close to the population of Tunisia as a whole, suggesting the unreliability of contemporary reports. There were, however, clearer indications of the relentlessness of the disease: during the month of April 1784, of 450 men in the northwest fort at Tabarca, only thirty survived the plague.[18]

Following the years of endemic plague (1794–1800), when limited outbreaks continued to take their toll, plague was absent for two decades. When it returned in epidemic form in 1818 the large-scale losses of the earlier epidemic were repeated. The usual exaggerated estimates by travelers are to be found: Rousseau stated that 50,000 perished in Tunis (nearly half the city's population).[19] In June 1818 Devoise thought that 30,000 had died in the city of Tunis; in September he raised his estimate to 40,000.[20] Gallico noted the exeptionally high mortality in the interior.[21] Valensi, extrapolating from a weekly register of Jewish mortality rates and from the daily mortality estimates compiled by Nyssen, reasoned that 30,000 deaths for the whole capital were not impossible: 'If Tunis numbered 120,000 inhabitants before the crisis, nearly a fourth of its population had disappeared. For the kingdom as a whole, the losses may well have been of the same order.'[22]

Did the apparent population decline continue after 1820 as a result of the later epidemics? During the nineteenth century Muslims and Europeans alike remarked that critical population declines were caused by them. The sources are monotonous in their pessimism: Muslim sources lament the golden age of Hamuda Bey (1782–1814); European sources criticize the indigenous government's failure to deal with the crises.

In the 1850s and 1860s Bin Diyaf and Bayram al-Khamis complained bitterly about the sad decline of prosperity and population during their lifetimes. Bin Diyaf gloomily claimed that during the epidemics 'half the people died from hunger and disease and this caused a big decrease in crops and livestock'.[23] Bayram al-Khamis commented that as a result of the 1867–8 epidemics 'the state is collapsing and is on its way to deterioration or extinction'.[24] In 1847 Pellissier de Reynaud stated that 'the Regency of Tunis is a cemetery of towns for which few tombs are provided with epitaphs'.[25] Meyebire predicted that it 'is a country that is gradually weakening, fatally, until the collapse arrives; in the middle of progress all around it, Tunisia will cease to be'.[26] It seems much of the lamentation by contemporaries was exaggerated for literary effect or political reasons. They were not writing to assist demographic historians of the 1980s. Officials such as Bin Diyaf and Bayram al-Khamis often wished to startle their compatriots into defensive reforms or to illustrate dramatically the misery of the events they witnessed. Some Europeans wished to emphasize the weakness of Tunisia in order to encourage or to justify European occupation.

Overall, however, demographic analyses do not indicate a population decline of this alleged magnitude in the nineteenth century. Mortality rates from the 1849–50 cholera epidemic, for example, can to some extent be reconstructed from the records kept by Abraham Lumbroso. According to his figures, there were about 7,600 deaths from cholera in Tunis and 56,000 for Tunisia as a whole.[27] He obtained his records from government officials, notables of the city of Tunis, European doctors, personnel who staffed the temporary hospitals, and tribal leaders. The estimates for the outlying regions were of course less accurate than those for the city. The crude death rate for Tunis, based on a population estimate of 150,000 inhabitants, was therefore 50/1,000, comparable with cholera figures from other Mediterranean cities of the time. For Tunisia as a whole, the crude death rate based on a total population of approximately 1.2 million

Fig. 8. Statistics compiled by Dr Lumbroso during the cholera epidemic of 1849–50

			Cases	Deaths
Tunis	Muslims	Men	3,700	1,800
		Women	4,800	2,100
	Jews	Men	4,100	1,900
		Women	3,500	1,500
			16,200	7,300
	Catholics	Men	300	230
		Women	175	70
			16,575	7,600

Towns in Province of Sousse (deaths)				
Sousse	Men	365	Women	282
Masakin		473		517
Qal'a Kabira		455		264
Jammal		402		169
Akuda		160		190
al-Hammam		56		71
Qal'a Saghira		67		61
al-Wardanin		93		131
al-Sahalin		65		66
al-Qasiba		75		85
al-Muskadin		46		42
Sidi al-Ahmar		32		23
Zawiyat Qundus		34		44
al-Manzal		83		59
Burgin		24		28
Sulayman		29		14
Bani Rabika		30		16
al-Kajas		14		16
al-Muradin		28		34
Bir al-Tayyib		13		14
Zawiyat Susa		83		79
Fariat		3		8
Sidi bu 'Ali		23		36
Hargla		51		61
Sakruna		29		28
Jardma		58		64
al-Zariba		49		36

	c. 5,278	5,278
Beja	4,000	1,700
Le Kef	4,800	2,000
Mountain tribes	10,000	5,000
Other nomadic tribes	21,000	13,000
Mateur	1,100	450
Bizerte	3,400	1,700
Portofarina and environs	900	370
Province of Djerid	18,000	8,000
Province of Gabes	5,700	2,000
Province of Nabeul	3,900	2,700
Province of Monastir	11,000	6,000
	83,800	48,198
Province of Sousse (cases)	18,000	
	101,800	

'Chart approximating cases of and deaths from cholera in the Regency of Tunis from 12 November 1849 to the end of August 1850, according to reports submitted by local authorities. They regret that exact numbers cannot be given because the nations which compose the total population resist registration (of births and deaths).'

was about 46/1,000. Lumbroso's fatality figures suggest the alarming medical inability to deal with the disease. According to Lumbroso, in Tunis 7,600 died out of 16,675 stricken – about 45 percent – while in the rest of Tunisia 48,198 persons died out of 101,800 stricken, or about 47 percent.[28] Lumbroso's list is only an estimate, however. There is no guarantee that all deaths were reported to the town authorities. Mortality rates for certain regions were estimates since most of the inhabitants were nomadic and far from the eye of officials. But even if the mortality figures are doubled, the result would not have been the dramatic population decline reported in the contemporary sources. Furthermore, figures for the European community of Tunis tend to corroborate Lumbroso's estimates: 113 Europeans were listed in the Catholic parish registers of Tunis as having died from cholera during June and July 1850, out of a total Catholic population of 9,150.[29]

The cholera epidemic of August 1856 was generally considered to have been less severe than that of 1849–50. Lumbroso did not publish records of it; there were two contemporary estimates. Dr Cotton reported that 130 Christians, 2,500 Jews, and 4,000 Muslims perished in the city of Tunis.[30] The Catholic parish registers list 46 deaths from cholera in August and September 1856.[31] Henri Dunant, the founder of the International Red Cross, visited Tunis in 1856. He commented favorably on the health of the city but reported that 200 Europeans had perished in the 1856 epidemic.[32]

Equally weak estimates exist for the epidemics of cholera and typhus of 1867–8. In a French consular report, 5,000 were reported dead of cholera in Tunis in two and a half months, and a total of about 18,000 to 20,000 for Tunisia. An additional 5,000 in Tunis were reported dead in the 1868 typhus epidemic. The Catholic parish register lists 114 dead from cholera from June to August 1867.[33]

The crude death rates from epidemic diseases must be correlated with other factors contributing to mortality rates. Population estimates are derived from population figures plus births, deaths, and migration in or out of the region. In the case of nineteenth-century Tunisia, the population was small, about one million after the plague epidemics of 1784–5 and 1818–20. It was also young; according to the partial census of 1862, more than 50 percent of the population was under twenty years of age.[34] Fertility rates were therefore high but so was mortality. Outmigration may have accounted for some of the pessimistic reports of population decline, but most people returned to their homes after the immediate crisis passed, after a few weeks or months. From reports of contemporaries, cholera struck persons of all ages rather than the demographically insignificant aged. The famine and other diseases such as tuberculosis, smallpox, typhoid fever, and dysenteries of course contributed to mortality rates. Yet none of these diseases appears to have been of a magnitude great enough to reverse the naturally high fertility rate. Despite the occurrence of epidemics and the reports of contemporaries, the population projection of 1.2 million corroborates the claim of population stability or slow population growth in Tunisia at the end of the nineteenth century.

Notes

Introduction

1 In L. Hirst, *The Conquest of Plague: A Study of the Evolution of Epidemiology* (Oxford, 1953); P. Ziegler, *The Black Death* (New York, 1969); J. Shrewsbury, *A History of Bubonic Plague in the British Isles* (Cambridge, 1970); J. Post, 'Famine, Mortality, and Epidemic Disease in the Process of Modernization', *Economic History Review*, 21, 1 (1976), 14–37.

2 J. May, *The Ecology of Human Disease* (New York, 1958); R. Pollitzer, *Cholera* (Geneva, 1959).

3 A. Briggs, 'Cholera and Society in the Nineteenth Century', *Past and Present*, 19 (1961), 76–96; N. Howard-Jones, 'Cholera Therapy in the Nineteenth Century', *Journal of the History of Medicine*, 27, 4 (October 1972), 373–95.

4 J. Snow, *Snow on Cholera* (New York, 1936), pp. 38–55.

5 A classic account of the history of typhus can be found in H. Zinsser, *Rats, Lice, and History* (New York, 1971).

6 G. Rosen, *A History of Public Health* (New York, 1958), pp. 64–9.

7 Frank, 'Tunis', p. 138. For further discussion of Avicennan medicine, see M. Shah, *The General Principles of Avicenna's Canon* (Karachi, 1966), pp. xii ff. For a concise survey in Arabic of Galenic knowledge of diseases and treatments, see al-Sabi Thabit Ibn Qurra, *The Book of al Dakhira* (*Kitab al-dakhira fi 'ilm al-tibb*), G. Sobhy, ed. (Cairo, 1928).

8 E. Bertherand, *Médecine et hygiène des Arabes* (Paris, 1855), pp. 406 and 469–70.

9 Husayn Ibn al-Mubarak, *al-Tajdid al-sahih* (Beirut, n.d.), pp. 134–5. See also Jalal al-Din al-Suyuti, 'Tibb ul-nabbi or Medicine of the Prophet', C. Elgood, trans., *Osiris* 14 (1962), 48–185. For hadiths on medicine, see J. Robson, *Mishkat al-masabih*, Vol. III (Lahore, 1964), pp. 945–54.

10 Indigenous medical practices have been extensively described. Accessible sources include: M. Hilton-Simpson, *Arab Medicine and Surgery: A Study of the Healing Art in Algeria* (London, 1922); J. Matignon, *L'Art médical à Tunis* (Paris, 1901); E. Doutté, *Magie et religion dans l'Afrique du nord* (Algiers, 1909), pp. 36–40; E. Westermarck, *Ritual and Belief in Morocco*, 2 vols. (London, 1926). In addition, most travelers' accounts contain at least a brief mention of medical practices. See, for example,

T. Shaw, *Travels and Observations Relating to Several Parts of Barbary and Levant* (Oxford, 1738), pp. 264–7; Peyssonnel, pp. 222–9.

11 Bertherand, *Médecine et hygiène*, p. 37.

12 *Ibid.*, pp. 37–8.

13 *Ibid.*

14 Westermarck, *Ritual and Belief*, pp. 262–301.

15 Bertherand, *Médecine et hygiène*, pp. 48–54.

16 V. Crapanzano, *The Hamadsha: A Study in Moroccan Ethnopsychiatry* (London, 1973).

17 For references to the medical explanations of such cures, see R. Brunel, *Essai sur la confrérie religieuse des 'Aissaoua au Maroc* (Paris, 1926), pp. xi–xvi and 138–40.

18 Brunel, *Essai sur la confrérie*, pp. 129–30 and 138–40. Many of these practices have been traced to West Africa, especially to the Hausa and Fulani. See also B. Greenwood, 'Ambiguity of Illness Classification in a Pluralistic Medical System: A Moroccan Example', MS (London, 1980); M. Gilsenan, *Saint and Sufi in Modern Egypt: An Essay in the Sociology of Religions* (New York, 1973).

19 Hirst, *The Conquest of Plague*, pp. 22 ff.

20 *Ibid.*, pp. 58–68.

21 L. King, *The Medical World of the Eighteenth Century* (Chicago, 1958), pp. 157 ff.

Chapter 1: Indigenous medicine against plague, 1780–1830

1 Ottoman military title which in Tunisia referred to the ruler. European sources usually used the term 'Regency of Tunis' for 'Tunisia' to emphasize its formal ties with the Ottoman Empire. Tunisian sources used the term *Mamlakata al-tunisiyya* (Kingdom of Tunis), or simply 'Tunis'.

2 T. Shaw, *Travels and Observations Relating to Several Parts of Barbary and Levant* (Oxford, 1738), p. 155.

3 *Kitab al-bashi*, pp. 186–7 ff.

4 *Ibid.*

5 A. Pellegrin, *Le Vieux Tunis: les noms des rues de la ville arabe* (Tunis, 1955), pp. 9 and 26.

6 Desfontaines, pp. 15–16.

7 Filippi counted eighteen hammams for men and fourteen for women in Tunis during the 1820s. C. Monchicourt, *Documents historiques sur la Tunisie: relations inédites de Nyssen, Filippi et Calligaris, 1788, 1829, 1834* (Paris, 1929), p. 82.

8 Peyssonnel, p. 14; Plantet, *Correspondance*, III, p. 50.

9 Frank, 'Tunis', pp. 136–7.

10 A.G.G.T., 794/5 (1234/1818–19 and 1271/1854–5).

11 Frank, 'Tunis', p. 137.

12 There were also earlier importations of European medical ideas. Husayn Khuja, a diplomat who made several voyages to Paris in the 1730s,

prepared a treatise on quinine using European source materials. J. Magnin, 'Médecine d'hier et médecins d'aujourd'hui', *Revue de l'institut des belles lettres arabes*, 80 (1957), 400 ff.

13 E. Bertherand, *Médecine et hygiène des Arabes* (Paris, 1855), pp. 18 and 24.

14 *Kitab al-bashi*, complete MSS Nos. 1236 and 1249, also photoplate, p. 38; Bin Diyaf, ii, p. 144; Magnin, 'Médecine d'hier', p. 399. Curillo wrote a study of the thermal waters of Tunis which was incorporated into Bayram al-Khamis's *al-Hammamat al-ma'daniya* (Cairo, 1906).

15 Masson, pp. 370 and 390; Plantet, *Correspondance*, iii, pp. 93 and 236–7.

16 Bin Diyaf, iii, p. 127.

17 Frank, 'Tunis', p. 75.

18 G. Brieger, *Medical America in the Nineteenth Century* (Baltimore, 1972), p. 94. For information on Ottoman physicians, see Adnan Adivar, *La Science chez les Turcs ottomans* (Paris, 1939), pp. 85–101, 127–30, 146–9, 159–60; and B. Lewis, *The Muslim Discovery of Europe* (New York, 1982), pp. 214–26. Adivar discusses numerous Muslim chief physicians and personal physicians to the sultans of the sixteenth to nineteenth centuries, and finds a preference for European physicians only in the second half of the eighteenth century. Lewis discusses Jewish–Italian physicians who practiced at the Ottoman court from the fifteenth century. In implying that European medicine had advanced over Islamic medicine by the fifteenth and sixteenth centuries, Lewis may predate the relative state of medical knowledge by some two centuries. The studies and sources cited by Adnan Adivar and Bedi Şehsuvaroğlu might help clarify the process of transition from Ottoman Islamic to European medicine in Istanbul.

19 A.G.G.T., 795/36 (May 1837).

20 M. al-Khuja, 'Wathiqa tarikhiya jalila', *al-Majallat al-zaytuna* (October 1939), 374–91.

21 A nasri purchased one loaf of bread in 1662. al-Khuja, 'Wathiqa tarikhiya', pp. 384–5. The term 'maristan' is derived from the pre-Islamic Persian *bimaristan*, a word that came into Arabic via Turkish. It was a correct term for 'hospital' in the seventeenth century but later became synonymous with 'mental asylum' or 'hospice for incurables', which is in fact what it became. The hospital was also known as 'Mustashfa 'Azzafin', after the suq for musical instruments in which it was located or, some said, after the band that played for the patients to help cure them. The maristan is now used as a shop in which carpets are sold. The original layout of the building is clearly the same as that described in the waqf document. al-Khuja, 'Wathiqa tarikhiya', p. 387.

22 B. Sfar, *Assistance publique musulmane en Tunis* (Tunis, 1896), pp. 11–12.

23 A.G.G.T., 700–5/5 and 700–5/6.

24 A.G.G.T., 700–5/1 and 700–5/3.

25 Monchicourt, *Documents historiques*, p. 38.

26 A.G.G.T., 700–5/4.

27 Bertherand, *Médecine et hygiène*, pp. 17–18.

28 Bin Diyaf, vi, p. 94.

29 Plantet, *Correspondance*, II, pp. 137–8.
30 Desfontaines, p. 56.
31 E. Bloch, *La Peste en Tunisie: aperçu historique et épidémiologique* (Tunis, 1929), pp. 8–9; *Kitab al-bashi*, 328.
32 A.G.G.T., 809/2.
33 Bin Diyaf, III, p. 20.
34 Masson (p. 600) includes commercial correspondence which dates the plague epidemic from 1883. al-Nasr (*Tarikh jirba* [Tunis, n.d.], pp. 25–6) dates it from 1784 to 1796, including the years of endemic plague.
35 Frank, 'Tunis', p. 130.
36 *Ibid.*
37 Peyssonnel, p. 228.
38 Abbé Poiret, *Voyage en Barbarie, ou lettres écrites de l'ancienne Numidia pendant les années de 1785 et 1786*, Vol. I (Paris, 1789), pp. 105–6.
39 M. Gandolphe, 'Notes inédites sur Tunisie en 1786 et sur son épidémie de peste en 1785, extraites du journal de Père Vicheret', *Revue tunisienne*, 25 (1918), 214–17.
40 Bin Diyaf, III, p. 14.
41 *Ibid.*, pp. 14–15.
42 Yusuf al-Sanusi al-Hasani, *Mujarrabat al-dirbiy al-kabir* (Tunis, n.d.), pp. 114–15.
43 Jalal al-Din al-Suyuti, 'Tibb ul-nabbi or Medicine of the Prophet', C. Elgood, trans., *Osiris*, 14 (1962), 149–51.
44 Jalal al-Din al-Suyuti, *al-Rahma fi al-tibb wa al-hikma* (Tunis, n.d.), pp. 84–6.
45 Da'ud al-Antaki, *Tadhkirat uli al-albab wa al-jami' al-ajab al-ujab* (Cairo, 1885–6), pp. 152–4. On Armenian earth, see M. Dols, *The Black Death in the Middle East* (Princeton, 1977), pp. 102ff, esp. p. 104.
46 Bibliothèque Nationale, Tunis, MS No. 1391.
47 Bertherand, *Médecine et hygiène*, p. 470.
48 Quoted in R. Neveu, 'L'Etat sanitaire de l'Afrique du nord pendant l'occupation arabo-turque', *Société française d'histoire de la médecine française*, 12 (1912), 517–18.
49 Peyssonnel, p. 228.
50 Gandolphe, 'Notes inédites', pp. 218–21.
51 Bloch, *La Peste en Tunisie*, pp. 2–4. Dr L. Frank had heard that olive oil porters were immune to plague and surmised that a treatment based on frictions might be effective. He suggested a series of experiments based on similar observations in other areas of the Mediterranean but the idea does not seem to have gained wide acceptance. Frank, 'Tunis', pp. 131–3.
52 J.N. Biraben, *Les Hommes et la peste en France et dans les pays européens et méditerranéens*, Vol. II (Paris, 1976), p. 12.
53 J. Marchika, *La Peste en Afrique septentrionale* (Algiers, 1927), p. 7. The funduq used by the French was constructed as a caravanserai in 1583 and was retained until 1860. G. Loth, *Le Peuplement italien en Tunisie et en Algérie* (Tunis, 1905), p. 1.

54 Gandolphe, 'Notes inédites', pp. 214–15.

55 Desfontaines, cited in Masson, p. 453. Jacques Berque informs me that he has observed similar actions in Morocco during cholera and typhus epidemics.

56 Poiret, *Voyage en Barbarie*, vol. I, pp. 105–6.

57 Plantet, *Correspondance*, III, DeVoise to Buchot (4 Thermidor, Year 11/22 July 1794), p. 238.

58 Neveu, 'L'Etat sanitaire', p. 509.

59 Valensi, *Fellahs tunisiens*, p. 270.

60 Bin Diyaf, III, pp. 127–8.

61 *Ibid.*, p. 128.

62 *Ibid.*

63 *Ibid.* For discussion of medieval Muslim interpretations of plague, see Dols, *The Black Death*; and J. Sublet, 'La Peste prise aux rets de la jurisprudence: le traité d'Ibn Hagar al 'Asqalani sur la peste', *Studia Islamica*, 33 (1971), 141–9.

64 Bin Diyaf, III, p. 129; A. Wensinck, *Concordance et indices de la tradition musulmane*, Vol. IV (Leiden, 1965), p. 91; J. Robson, *Mishkat al-masabih*, Vol. III (Lahore, 1964), pp. 955–6.

65 L. Valensi, *Le Maghreb avant la prise d'Alger* (Paris, 1969), p. 73.

66 L. Valensi, 'Islam et capitalisme: production et commerce des chechias en Tunisie et en France aux XVIIIe et XIXe siècles', *Revue d'histoire moderne et contemporaine*, 16 (1969), 376–400.

67 R. Limam, 'Siyasa hamuda basha al-husayni fi al-mahal al-tijari', *Revue d'histoire maghrebine*, 2 (July 1974), 85–6.

68 Bin Diyaf, VII, p. 96.

69 Frank, 'Tunis', pp. 78–83; Plantet, *Correspondance*, III, letter of 30 October 1808.

70 *Kitab al-bashi*, pp. 186–7ff.

71 Valensi, *Fellahs tunisiens*, pp. 304–15.

72 Masson, p. 502.

73 *Ibid.*, p. 596.

74 *Ibid.*

75 Valensi, 'Islam et capitalisme', pp. 396–9.

76 L. Valensi, 'Calamités démographiques en Tunisie et en Méditerranée orientale aux XVIIIe et XIXe siècles', *Annales*, *E.S.C.*, 6 (November–December 1969), 1548–9. The merchant ships were small brigs weighing about 200 tons. In preceding years the number of ships leaving Marseilles for Tunis per year was as follows:

1776	16	1780	18	1784	23
1777	17	1781	23	1785	28
1778	15	1782	29	1786	42
1779	10	1783	18	1787	82

Masson, pp. 598–601.

77 M.H. Cherif, 'Les Domaines de l'histoire: l'expansion européenne et difficultés tunisiennes de 1815 à 1830', *Annales, E.S.C.*, 3, 25 (1970), 714–15.

78 Plantet, *Correspondance*, III, pp. 127–8.

79 Cherif, 'Les Domaines de l'histoire', pp. 719–22.

80 Valensi (*Le Maghreb avant la prise*, pp. 62–9) suggests that European privateers in the seventeenth and eighteenth centuries intentionally prevented the development of a Muslim merchant marine and that this forced the beys to counterattack in self-defense. P. Grandchamp, *Documents relatifs aux corsaires tunisiens, 1777–1824* (Tunis, 1925) contains a list of passports issued to Tunisian corsairs from 1792 to 1824.

81 M. Bdira, *Relations internationales et sous-développement: la Tunisie, 1857–1864* (Uppsala, 1978), pp. 30–1.

82 Bin Diyaf, III, p. 129.

83 Valensi, 'Calamités démographiques', pp. 1556–8. For further information, see Appendix C.

84 Cherif, 'Les Domaines de l'histoire', pp. 723–4.

85 *Ibid.*, pp. 726–7.

86 *Ibid.*, pp. 730–7.

87 See also the conclusions of Cherif concerning the secondary role of the plague epidemics, in *ibid.*, pp. 722–30.

Chapter 2: Cholera in an age of European economic expansion, 1830–58

1 M. Bdira, *Relations internationales et sous-developpement: la Tunisie, 1857–1864* (Uppsala, 1978), p. 31.

2 A.G.G.T., 809/2, Husayn Bey to Mathieu de Lesseps (7 Rabi' Ithani 1244/17 December 1828).

3 Here the bey was referring to his religious belief in divine omnipotence, which had perhaps led to his antiquarantine stance during the earlier plague epidemic. He may have resolved his initial uncertainty regarding quarantining in accord with a well-known hadith cited in Bukhari's *Sahih*: 'A man asked the Prophet Muhammad if he should separate his sick camel from the rest of the herd. The Prophet told him to separate the camel, but added that this might not save the others because the sickness had come to the first one from somewhere. And who brought the epidemic to the first?' Husayn Ibn al-Mubarak, *al-Tajdid al-sahih* (Beirut, n.d.), p. 135; A. Wensinck, *Concordance et indices de la tradition musulmane*, Vol. IV (Leiden, 1965), p. 157; J. Robson, *Mishkat al-masabih*, Vol. III (Lahore, 1964), p. 955.

4 A.G.G.T., 809/5, Husayn Bey to Mathieu de Lesseps (4 Dhu al-Hijja 1247/5 May 1832); A.G.G.T., 809/3, Husayn Bey to Thomas Reade (30 Rabi' Ithani 1247/8 October 1831).

5 L. Chevalier, *La Choléra: la première épidémie du XIXe siècle* (La Roche-sur-Yon, 1958), p. 134.

6 A.G.G.T., 798/23, minutes of first meeting of Sanitary Council [also called 'Consiglio Sanitario' in Italian or *majlis al-tahaffuz* in Arabic] (19 November 1835). See J. Montague, 'Notes on Medical Organization in Nineteenth Century Tunisia: A Preliminary Analysis of the Materials on Public Health and Medicine in the Dar el Bey in Tunis', *Medical History*, 17, 1 (January 1973), 75–82, for a translation of this document into English and a description of the contents of the Tunisian archives that pertain to matters of public health.

7 A.G.G.T., 798–822 contain the bulk of the correspondence of the council, though additional materials are found in other dossiers.

8 A.G.G.T., 798/23. Similar councils were set up in Syria (M. Ma'oz, *Ottoman Reform in Syria and Palestine*, 1840–1861 [Oxford, 1968], p. 167); in Beirut (C. Issawi, 'British Trade and the Rise of Beirut, 1830–1860', *International Journal of Middle East Studies*, 8, 1 [January 1977], 92–3); in Tangiers (L. Vaidon, *Tangier: A Different Way* [Metuchen, N.J., 1977], p. 57); and in Egypt (L. Kuhnke, 'Resistance and Response to Modernization: Preventive Medicine and Social Control in Egypt' [Ph.D. dissertation, Chicago, 1971], pp. 70ff).

9 A.G.G.T., 799/29, ten articles of quarantine procedures plus provisions for privateering ships (which were to undergo quarantine 'like the others' at La Goulette). A.G.G.T., 799/30, conditions for quarantine; the fifth condition concerns privateer ships.

10 F.O., Lloyd to Hay (23 January 1836).

11 L. Chevalier, *Classes laborieuses et classes dangereuses à Paris pendant la première moitié du XIXe siècle* (Paris, 1958).

12 It is impossible to know if quarantines were responsible for preventing the spread of cholera to Tunisia, since many other epidemics had come and were to come from the outside despite the practice of quarantining. This does not rule out the possibility that a series of effectively administered quarantines might have controlled transmission, although this is unlikely given the ease of cordon evasion. Individuals or boats frequently escaped the watch of quarantine officials, not only in Tunisia but elsewhere. If it were possible to control human traffic, transmission could theoretically have been avoided.

13 A.G.G.T., 798/26, Sanitary Council to Ahmad Bey (9 March 1845).

14 F. Lovy, 'Notes sur la vie médicale à Tunis avant l'occupation', *La Tunisie médicale*, special edn (May 1931), 209–17; E. Molco, 'L'Art médical en Tunisie avant le protectorat', *La Tunisie Médicale*, special edn (May 1931), 184–206; and H. Dunant, *La Régence de Tunis* (Tunis, 1975), pp. 229–30. Dunant gives a list of about twenty European doctors whom he found practicing in Tunisia in 1856.

15 A.G.G.T., 809/28, Ahmad Bey to amir al-liwa' of Sousse and other port officials (10 Shawwal 1264/9 September 1848).

16 *Ibid.*

17 A.G.G.T., 813/133, Mahmuda, kahiya of La Goulette, to Ahmad Bey (26 Dhu al-Qada 1265/13 October 1849).

18 F.O., 102 (18 Ramadan 1265/7 August 1849).
19 A.G.G.T., 799/70, regulations issued 4 October 1849.
20 Lumbroso, *Cenni sul cholera*, p. 37.
21 A.G.G.T., 708/81, Sanitary Council to Ahmad Bey (November 1849).
22 Lumbroso, *Cenni sul cholera*, pp. 37ff.
23 *Ibid.*
24 *Ibid.*, p. 39.
25 A.G.G.T., 799/84, Sanitary Council to Ahmad Bay (2 December 1849).
26 Lumbroso, *Cenni sul cholera*, p. 42.
27 A.G.G.T., 799/85, Sanitary Council to Ahmad Bey (6 December 1849);
   Lumbroso, *Cenni sul cholera*, pp. 55ff.
28 A.G.G.T., 799/85, Sanitary Council to Ahmad Bey (6 December 1849).
29 Lumbroso, *Cenni sul cholera*, pp. 51–4.
30 *Ibid.*, pp. 56–7.
31 A.G.G.T., 799/86, Sanitary Council to Ahmad Bey (14 December 1849).
32 *Ibid.*
33 Both books were published in Marseilles, in 1850 and 1860 respectively,
   and can be found in the National Library of Medicine in Bethesda,
   Maryland.
34 Bin Diyaf, IV, p. 129.
35 Lumbroso, *Cenni sul cholera*, pp. 61–2.
36 Bin Diyaf, IV, pp. 131–2.
37 Lumbroso, *Cenni sul cholera*, pp. 70–4.
38 J. Guyon, 'Lettre sur l'état de choléra dans la régence de Tunis', *Gazette
   médicale de Paris*, 3rd ser., 5 (1850), 401.
39 Lumbroso, *Cenni sul cholera*, pp. 43–50.
40 Bin Diyaf, IV, p. 130.
41 *Ibid.*, VIII (*tabaqat*), pp. 74–5; Lumbroso, *Cenni sul cholera*, pp. 134–5.
42 Lumbroso, *Cenni sul cholera*, pp. 54–5.
43 *Ibid.*
44 Guyon, 'Lettre sur l'état', p. 401.
45 Bin Diyaf, IV, p. 133.
46 *Ibid.*, pp. 129–30.
47 *Ibid.*, p. 130.
48 *Ibid.*, pp. 134–5.
49 Lumbroso, *Cenni sul cholera*, pp. 140–1.
50 *Ibid.*, p. 230.
51 *Ibid.*, pp. 135–6.
52 A.G.G.T., 800/5, Sanitary Council to Ahmad Bey (13 March 1850).
53 A.G.G.T., 795/122, Clot Bey to Ahmad Bey (1854).
54 Lumbroso, *Cenni sul cholera*, pp. 152–3 and 179.
55 The French government had given Ahmad the *Minos* on his return from
   his state visit to Paris in 1846.
56 Bin Diyaf, IV, p. 131.
57 Lumbroso, *Cenni sul cholera*, pp. 175–6.
58 *Ibid.*, p. 228.

59 *Ibid.*, p. 230.
60 Bin Diyaf, IV, pp. 133–4.
61 Bibliothèque Nationale, Tunis, MS No. 16511.
62 Bin Diyaf, IV, pp. 134–5.
63 Lumbroso, *Cenni sul cholera*, p. 231.
64 *Ibid.*, pp. 218–19.
65 *Ibid.*; M. Ladjimi, 'L'Empirisme médical chez les musulmans tunisiens', doct. d'état, médecine (Lyon, 1920).
66 E. Bertherand, *Médecine et hygiène des Arabes* (Paris, 1855), p. 431.
67 *Ibid.*, p. 55.
68 Lumbroso, *Cenni sul cholera*, pp. 214–18.
69 N. Howard-Jones, 'Cholera Therapy in the Nineteenth Century', *Journal of the History of Medicine*, 27, 4 (October 1972), 373–95.
70 B. Şehsuvaroğlu, *Tarihi kolera salginlare ve oslanle turkleri* (Istanbul, 1954), pp. 286ff.
71 At least three copies of this manuscript are to be found in the Bibliothèque Nationale in Tunis. They are MSS Nos. 1219, 1391, and 19823. There is at least one copy in the Zahiriya Library in Damascus (S. Hamarneh, *Fihris makhtutat dar al-kutub al-zahiriyya: al-tibb wa al-saydala* [Damascus, 1969]).
72 A.G.G.T., 817/108, 'Amr al-'Ayadi to Isma'il Sahib al-Taba' (1 Dhu al-Qada 1272/4 July 1856); A.G.G.T., 817/119, 'Amr al-'Ayadi to Isma'il Sahib al-Taba' (27 Muharram 1272/10 October 1855); A.G.G.T., 817/109, 'Amr al-'Ayadi to Isma'il Sahib al-Taba' (29 Muharram 1272/12 October 1855); A.G.G.T., 817/117, 'Amr al-'Ayadi to Isma'il Sahib al-Taba' (18 Safar al-Khayr 1272/31 October 1855).
73 A.G.G.T., 800/10, Sanitary Council to Muhammad Bey (21 July 1856); Bin Diyaf, IV, pp. 211 and 267.
74 W. McNeill, *Plagues and Peoples: A History* (New York, 1976), p. 264.
75 A. Lumbroso, *Lettres médico-statistiques sur la régence de Tunis* (Marseilles, 1860), p. 117.
76 *Ibid.*
77 *Ibid.*
78 J. Ganiage, *Les Origines du protectorat français en Tunisie* (Paris, 1959), pp. 158–60; Molco, 'L'Art médical', pp. 185–90. Molco says he was honored by the affection of the sovereigns he served and aided those who sought his assistance without consideration of nationality, religion, or social class.
79 Bin Diyaf, IV, Section 1, reign of Ahmad Bey.
80 A.G.G.T., 800/43, Sanitary Council to Ahmad Bey (25 July 1854).
81 A.G.G.T., 800/58, Sanitary Council to Ahmad Bey (9 October 1856).
82 A.G.G.T., 800/77, Sanitary Council to Ahmad Bey (9 March 1855).
83 Bin Diyaf, IV, pp. 136–7. For discussion of cholera's demographic effects, see Appendix C.
84 *Ibid.*, pp. 150–5. For a complete account of the machinations of Bin 'Ayad, see L. C. Brown, *The Tunisia of Ahmad Bey*, 1837–1855 (Princeton, 1974), Ch. 10.

85 Bin Diyaf, IV, pp. 224–8.
86 *Ibid.*, p. 255; M. Mabrouk, 'La municipalité de Tunis avant et sous la colonisation', *La Presse* (Tunis, 13 May 1975), p. 3.
87 Bin Diyaf, IV, p. 264.

Chapter 3: Cholera, typhus, and economic collapse, 1858–70

1 For further information on the 'ahd al-aman, see A. Laroui, *L'Histoire du Maghreb: un essai de synthèse* (Paris, 1970), pp. 289–90; Bin Diyaf, IV, pp. 131ff; and M. Bdira, *Relations internationales et sous-developpement: la Tunisie, 1857–1864* (Uppsala, 1978), pp. 51ff.
2 Bin Diyaf, V, pp. 22–3ff.
3 Ganiage, *Origines*, pp. 54–60.
4 Ganiage, *Origines*, pp. 211–16.
5 In a consular letter of 1863, De Beauval estimated that the land under cultivation had fallen from 60,000 measures under Muhammad Bey to 40,000 under Sadiq Bey (1 measure = approximately 10 hectares). Villet, a member of the International Finance Commission that managed Tunisian finances after 1868, estimated the amount of land under cultivation in 1837 to be about 1 million hectares. The increase in agricultural exports along with the shrinkage of land under cultivation was a contributing factor to the famine of 1865–7. Ganiage, *Origines*, pp. 175 and 223. See also Bin Diyaf, V, pp. 124–31.
6 Bin Diyaf, V, pp. 121ff and 184–5; B. Slama, *L'Insurrection de 1864 en Tunisie* (Tunis, 1967), pp. 101–38.
7 *Safwat al-i'tibar*, p. 34.
8 Bin Diyaf, VI, p. 89.
9 *Ibid.*
10 Ganiage, *Origines*, p. 304.
11 Bin Diyaf, VI, pp. 86–7.
12 *Safwat al-i'tibar*, p. 35.
13 Ganiage, *Origines*, p. 46. There were about 7,000 Maltese, 4,000 Italians (mostly Sicilians), 250 Greeks, and 200 to 300 French nationals in mid-nineteenth-century Tunisia. During the 1860s and 1870s, the number of Italians increased rapidly. There were only about 700 to 800 French nationals in Tunisia in 1881.
14 The articles of the International Sanitation Convention held in 1861 in Istanbul were printed in Arabic in *Ra'id al-tunisi* (5 Muharram 1283/19 April 1886). A.G.G.T., 803/92 is a copy of these regulations.
15 A.G.G.T., 817/129, Haydar Agha to Rustam, wazir al-'amala (Dhu al-Qada 1282/February–March 1866).
16 A.G.G.T., 817/128, Mustafa, 'amil of Bizerte and Ghar al-Milh, to Mustafa Khaznadar, wazir al-akbar (19 Rabi' al-Awal 1282/12 August 1865).
17 The village was so named after immigrants from Andalusian Spain who had settled there in the seventeenth century.

18 Ferrini, *Intorno al cholera*, p. 6.

19 *Ibid.*, pp. 6ff.

20 A.G.G.T., 817/104, Salih b. 'Ali, 'amil of Bizerte and Ghar al-Milh, to Rustam (15 Dhu al-Hijja 1283/21 April 1867).

21 A.G.G.T., 817/104, Hathar b. Shaykh Husayn, shaykh of Qal'at al-Andalus, to Salim, ra'is al-dhabityya (25 Dhu al-Hijja 1283/1 May 1867).

22 Gustave Nachtigal was later to write his famous account of his explorations in the Sudan, *Sahara und Soudan* (Berlin, 1879); English translation by A. Fisher and H. Fisher (Berkeley, 1971). Nachtigal had originally settled in Tunisia for reasons of health but because of the famine and cholera of 1867, he departed for the Sudan. He later returned to Tunis as consul general of Germany.

23 Ferrini, *Intorno al cholera*, p. 6.

24 A.G.G.T., 817/101, Hathar b. Shaykh Husayn to Salim (27 Dhu al-Hijja 1283/3 May 1867).

25 A.G.G.T., 817/100, Salih b. 'Ali to Rustam (27 Muharram 1284/31 May 1867).

26 A.G.G.T., 817/99. The price of wheat was twenty-seven copper riyals, and barley was eleven (12 Safar al-Khayr 1284/15 June 1867).

27 A.G.G.T., 817/61 (20 Safar al-Khayr 1284/23 June 1867)

28 *Ibid.*

29 *Ibid.*

30 *Ibid.*

31 A.G.G.T., 817/92, Salih b. 'Ali to Rustam (23 Safar al-Khayr 1284/26 June 1867) and A.G.G.T., 817/96 (24 Safar al-Khayr 1284/ 27 June 1867). The sickness was reported to be abating in Bizerte, where only 22 persons died on Monday. But in a letter dated two days later, it was said to have increased again (A.G.G.T., 817/97).

32 A.G.G.T., 817/97, Salih b. 'Ali to Rustam (10 Rabi' al-Awal 1284/12 July 1867); A.G.G.T., 817/98, Salih b. 'Ali to Rustam (17 Safar al-Khayr 1284/20 June 1867). In a letter dated a month later, Salih mentioned a heat wave which was damaging fruit and corn.

33 Bin Diyaf, VI, p. 91.

34 Ferrini, *Intorno al cholera*, p. 7.

35 A.G.G.T., 817/89 and 817/90, bu Bakr b. Salam, kahiya khalifa, to Rustam (2 Safar al-Khayr 1284/5 June 1867).

36 A.G.G.T., 817/89; A.G.G.T., 803/78 (11 June 1867); A.G.G.T., 817/24, bu Bakr b. Salam to Rustam (20 Safar al-Khayr 1284/23 June 1867); A.G.G.T., 817/29, Penna to Mustafa Khaznadar (20 Safar al-Khayr 1284/23 June 1867).

37 A.G.G.T., 817/52, bu Bakr b. Salam to Rustam; A.G.G.T., 817/112, Salah al-Mazali, khalifa of Monastir, to Mustafa Khaznadar (23 Safar al-Khayr 1284/26 June 1867).

38 A.G.G.T., 817/3–77 *passim*. Among the Europeans who perished in Sousse was the vice-consul of France (A.G.G.T., 817/9).

39 A.G.G.T., 817/7, khalifa of Sousse to Rustam (12 June 1867).

40 Ferrini, *Intorno al cholera*, p. 8.
41 Bin Diyaf, VI, pp. 91ff.
42 Ferrini, *Intorno al cholera*, pp. 8ff.
43 The disease had appeared there sporadically since early April. The mufti of Beja had been one of the first to perish. A.G.G.T., 817/105 (12 Dhu al-Hijja 1283/18 April 1867).
44 Bin Diyaf, VI, p. 91.
45 A.G.G.T., 817/145, 'Ali al-Sasi, amir al-liwa' and 'amil of the Djerid, to Mustafa Khaznadar (19 Rabi' al-Awal 1284/21 July 1867). al-Sasi complained that he had gone to Nefta to avoid the disease but that while he was sleeping there, some of his staff had escaped to Tunis.
46 A.G.G.T., 817/143, 'Ali al-Sasi to Muhammad al-'Aziz bu 'Attur, bash katib and wazir al-mal (19 Rabi' al-Awal 1284/21 July 1867).
47 A.G.G.T., 817/107, 'Ali al-Sasi to Rustam (3 Rabi' Ithani 1284/5 September 1867). He said that several high-ranking officers had died, as had the qadi of Tozeur. The 'amil said there was no cure for the sickness.
48 A.G.G.T., 817/115, 'Amr b. Katib to Isma'il Sahib al-Taba' (14 Rabi' al-Awal 1284/16 July 1867).
49 See Chapter 2.
50 A.G.G.T., 817/80, minutes of Sanitary Council (8 July 1867). The council asked the government to provide a better lazaret than that on the island of Zimbala and to rebuild the one at Sfax, which had been destroyed during the 1864 insurrection. The council also asked the bey to place some of his own ships at the disposal of travelers so that they could spend the week or two of quarantine in greater comfort.
51 A.G.G.T., 803/79, Werry to Sadiq Bey (17 June 1867). The message was sent on behalf of the consuls of England, Italy, Austria, and Sweden. They complained that the cordon at Hammam Lif only prevented those already sick from entering Tunis. They noted that the disease took twelve days to appear and advised that all persons and caravans should be stopped to insure the safety of the capital.
52 Ferrini, *Intorno al cholera*, p. 11.
53 Bin Diyaf, VI, p. 91.
54 *Safwat al-i'tibar*, p. 35.
55 Lumbroso, *Cenni sul cholera*, p. 72.
56 Husayn Sharif was president of the Municipal Council in the early 1860s. He was exiled a few months after the events of 1867 for his political opposition to Mustafa Khaznadar. He returned in 1870 and became minister of education in 1874 with the accession of Khayr al-Din.
57 Mustafa Khaznadar (George Kalkias Stravelakis) was born on the island of Chios in 1817. The nephews were sons of a brother who had remained in Chios in 1821 (Ganiage, *Origines*, pp. 90ff). Bin Diyaf stated that he had learned of his expenditure from a receipt he had seen on the fifteenth page of a state treasury register kept by Khaznadar (Bin Diyaf, VI, p. 92).
58 Bin Diyaf, VI, p. 92.
59 F.O., 102/80, Werry to Stanley (8 July 1867).

60 Ferrini, *Intorno al cholera*, pp. 12–14.

61 *Ibid.*, pp. 24–66. For a medical discussion of such remedies, see N. Howard-Jones, 'Cholera Therapy in the Nineteenth Century', *Journal of the History of Medicine*, 27, 4 (October 1972), 373–95.

62 F.O., 102/80, Werry to Stanley (8 July 1867). In the letter, Werry commented that 'although the disease has not as yet reached the magnitude of the 1856 epidemic among the city's 150,000 inhabitants, a much greater panic has been caused eliciting a considerable emigration to Europe by those who possess the means'.

63 A.G.G.T., 803/88, minutes of Sanitary Council (5 July 1867). The council stated in this letter that according to a religious custom, Muslims waited two or three days to bury their dead, i.e., too long, and that the Hebrews buried their dead too soon. The observations by the council were not only impossible to enforce, but also inaccurate. The *Shari'a* (Islamic law) called for immediate interment and Jewish families often held watches for a few days.

64 A.G.G.T., 803/101, minutes of Sanitary Council (3 September 1867).

65 *Ra'id al-tunisi* (20 Jumada Ithani 1284/19 October 1867), p. 1.

66 C. Dessort, *L'Histoire de la ville de Tunis* (Algiers, 1924), p. 121. The year of famine became known as *bu barak* (father of kneeling).

67 Ganiage, *Origines*, p. 310.

68 Bin Diyaf, VI, p. 104.

69 *Ibid.*

70 A.G.G.T., 803/48, minutes of Sanitary Council (14 February 1868). The Sanitary Council continued to issue clean patents to ships departing from Tunis in accordance with the International Convention of Paris, 1852.

71 A.G.G.T., 803/140, Werry to Mustafa Khaznadar (9 February 1868).

72 *Ibid.* The theory that typhus germs could change into plague germs was a commonly held one. Though modern science has proven the theory fallacious, the idea that unsanitary conditions contributed to the spread of disease was of course perfectly correct.

73 A.G.G.T., 803/76, minutes of Sanitary Council (11 December 1868).

74 An epizootic (epidemic of animals), primarily of cattle, was currently raging. This disease was not identified at the time and was associated by contemporaries with the cholera and typhus epidemics. F.O., 102/80 (August 1867); A.G.G.T., 803/138, Sanitary Council to Mustafa Khaznadar (20 January 1868); A.G.G.T., 803/44, minutes of Sanitary Council (12 February 1868).

75 A.G.G.T., 803/146, Werry to Mustafa Khaznadar (14 February 1868).

76 A.G.G.T., 803/179, minutes of Sanitary Council (23 December 1868); A.G.G.T., 803/148 (14 February 1868); A.G.G.T., 803/159 (15 April 1868).

77 Now rue Mongi Slim; A.G.G.T., 803/159.

78 A.G.G.T., 803/145, Mustafa Khaznadar to Werry (22 Shawwal 1284/16 February 1868).

79 Bin Diyaf, VI, p. 104.
80 *Ibid.*, p. 105.
81 A.G.G.T., 803 contains an undated list of articles entitled 'Qanun li tanzim sharawi' hadra Tunis' (laws for the cleaning of the streets of Tunis).
82 Bin Diyaf, VI, p. 104. Bin Diyaf provided the names of five of the assessed notables.
83 *Safwat al-i'tibar*, p. 37.
84 *Ibid.*, p. 36.
85 *Ibid.*
86 *Ibid.*
87 Bin Diyaf, VI, pp. 96–102 and 114; F.O., 102, Werry to Stanley (14 May 1867, 17 September 1867, 5 October 1867).
88 Bin Diyaf, VI, p. 105.
89 For a detailed account of the financial crisis of 1864–8, see Ganiage, *Origines*, Chs. 6 and 7, also chart, p. 349.
90 Middle East Centre, St Antony's College, Oxford, Richard Wood papers, Richard Wood to Edmund Hammond, Foreign Office (29 October 1867). For further discussion of this affair, see Ganiage, *Origines*, pp. 311–12.
91 Ganiage, *Origines*, pp. 370ff.

Chapter 4: Colonization and collapse of Arab medical institutions

1 A.G.G.T., 794/8 and 794/3.
2 A.G.G.T., 794/4.
3 A.G.G.T., 794/1.
4 A.G.G.T., 794/20.
5 A.G.G.T., 794/9.
6 A.G.G.T., 793/1, 794/2, 794/6.
7 Translation and illustration of the nominating letter in N. Gallagher, 'The Arab Medical Organization in Nineteenth-Century Tunisia', *Revue d'histoire maghrebine*, 4 (July 1975), 145–9.
8 Under a nineteenth-century French medical regulation, a student who had completed the course work but had not submitted the required thesis was awarded the title of officer of health and allowed to practice.
9 A.G.G.T., 795/123 (21 Rabi' Ithani 1293/16 April 1876).
10 B. Dinguizli, 'Aperçu rétrospectif sur l'exercice de la profession médicale et de l'assistance médicale en Tunisie avant l'occupation française dans ce pays', *La Tunisie médicale*, special edn (May 1931), 181–3.
11 E. Molco, 'L'Art médical en Tunisie avant le protectorat', *La Tunisie médicale*, special edn (May 1931), 199–200.
12 A.G.G.T., 794/18 (4 September 1977).
13 Ganiage, *Origines*, pp. 558–9.
14 A.G.G.T., 795/122.
15 Ganiage, *Origines*, pp. 160–1. Certain French doctors also played a political role. Clement César, a doctor who served Sadiq Bey, was charged with a

diplomatic mission to the court of Napoleon III, following the absconding of Mustafa Khaznadar in 1873. F. Lovy, 'Notes sur la vie médicale à Tunis avant l'occupation', *La Tunisie médicale*, special edn (May 1931), 210.

16 A.G.G.T., 795/129 (2 January 1876) (in Arabic); A.G.G.T., 817/124 (1 January 1877) (in French).

17 Lumbroso, Castelnuovo, Vignale, Mascaro, and Spezzafumo, in that order, occupied the position of chief physician at court from 1835 to 1892, after which time Ottian Bonnet was appointed. Molco, 'L'Art médicale', p. 184.

18 Ganiage, *Origines*, pp. 465–6.

19 Khayr al-Din al-Tunisi, *The Surest Path*, L.C. Brown, trans. (Cambridge, 1967), pp. 141ff.

20 *La Presse* (Tunis, 13 May 1975), p. 3. A list of members of the Municipal Council's committee appeared in *Nuzhat al-khayriyya*, the government almanac (Tunis, 1296/1878–9).

21 A.G.G.T., 817/166 (1 Rabi' al-Awal 1289/9 May 1873); A.G.G.T., 814/11 (4 Jumada al-Akhira 1291/19 July 1874); L. Hirst, *The Conquest of Plague : A Study of the Evolution of Epidemiology* (Oxford, 1953), p. 74.

22 *Ra'id al-tunisi* (26 Dhu al-Qada 1286/27 February 1870).

23 The charter of the new hospital was published in *Ra'id al-tunisi* (13 Safar al-Khayr 1296/6 February 1879).

24 A.G.G.T., 807 (8 January 1880, 11 June 1880, 30 December 1880, 14 March 1881, 6 November 1882).

25 A.G.G.T., 822/89–90 (30 September 1884, 3 October 1884).

26 *Journal officiel tunisien* (5 March 1885), pp. 519–23.

27 *Ibid.*

28 A.G.G.T., 807/28 (5 September 1884).

29 M. Ladjimi, 'L'Empirisme médical chez les musulmans tunisiens', doct. d'état, médicine (Lyon, 1920), pp. 9–12.

30 J. Magnin, 'Médecine d'hier et médecins d'aujourd'hui', *Revue de l'institut des belles lettres arabes*, 80 (1957), 408–16.

31 F. Lovy, 'L'Hôpital Sadiki de 1893 à 1902', *La Tunisie médicale*, special edn (May 1931), 225–32.

32 Docteur Perussel, 'L'Assistance des psychopathes en Tunisie', *La Tunisie médicale*, special edn (May 1931), 277.

33 M. Gandolphe, 'Premiers hôpitaux français en Tunisie', *La Tunisie médicale*, special edn (May 1931), 167–70.

34 A.G.G.T., letter to Monsieur le Délégué à la Résidence Générale de la République Française, Tunis (6 January 1912); P. Johnson, 'A Sufi Shrine in Tunisia', Ph.D. dissertation (Berkeley, 1979). For a discussion of current medical practices, see C. H. Klein, 'Changing Health Beliefs and Practices in an Urban Setting: A Tunisian Example', Ph.D. dissertation (New York, 1975).

35 E. Bertherand, *Médecine et hygiène des Arabes* (Paris, 1855), pp. 547–54.

36 F. Gomma, *L'Assistance médicale en Tunisie : essai sur l'histoire de la médecine et de l'hygiène publique dans la régence* (Tunis, 1904), p. 10; Ladjimi, 'L'Empirisme médical', pp. 9–12. Nicolo Converti was a leader

of the nineteenth-century Tunisian labor movement and an internationally known anarchist; he practiced medicine in Tunisia under this law. After a brief imprisonment in Italy and suspension from medical school, he emigrated to Tunis in 1887, where he played an active role in the establishment of free medical services for poor workers. C. Liauzu, 'Les Libertaires en Tunisie', *Cahiers de Tunisie*, 21 (1973), 157–82.

37 R. Neveu, 'L'Etat sanitaire de l'Afrique du nord pendant l'occupation arabo-turque', *Société française d'histoire de la médecine française*, 12 (1912), 519.

Appendix A: Waqf (hubus) document for the maristan of Tunis

1 Translated from copy edited and published by M. al-Khuja in *al-Majallat al-zaytuna* (October 1939), 385–8. Abu 'Abd Allah Muhammad Basha was known as Hamuda Basha al-Muradi.

Appendix C: Epidemics and population trends

1 L.C. Brown, *The Tunisia of Ahmad Bey, 1837–1855* (Princeton, 1974), pp. 376–7; Valensi, *Fellahs tunisiens*, p. 13.

2 Pellissier de Reynaud, quoted in M. Rouissi, 'Villes, villages, et tribus de Tunisie à la fin du XIXe siècle', unpublished paper, pp. 3–4.

3 J. Ganiage, 'La Population de la Tunisie vers 1860: essai d'évaluation d'après les registres fiscaux', *Population*, 21, 5 (September–October 1966), 868.

4 M. Seklani, *La Population da la Tunisie* (Tunis, 1974), p. 19. Ganiage wonders whether a fourth or a fifth of the population perished during these years ('La Population de la Tunisie', p. 867).

5 I would like to thank Ned Levine, Urban Planning, U.C.L.A., for his assistance with these estimates.

6 Lumbroso, *Cenni sul cholera*, p. 16.

7 F.O., 102/80, Werry to Stanley.

8 Brown, *The Tunisia of Ahmad Bey*, pp. 375–8.

9 A. Raymond, 'Signes urbains et étude de la population des grandes villes arabes à l'époque ottomane', *Bulletin d'études orientales*, 27 (1974), 183–93. Most Islamic–Mediterranean cities had about one hammam per 3,000 to 4,000 inhabitants; Raymond based his estimate on Filippi's count of 32 hammams in Tunis in 1832. See C. Monchicourt, *Documents historiques sur la Tunisie: relations inédites de Nyssen, Filippi et Calligaris, 1788, 1829, 1834* (Paris, 1929), p. 82.

10 A. Lézine, *Deux villes d'Ifriqiyya* (Paris, 1971), pp. 164–9.

11 A. Loir, 'Démographie–statistique de la population de Tunis', *Revue tunisienne*, 19 (1898), 384 – 54.

12 Ganiage, 'Population de la Tunisie', p. 858.

13 P. Sebag, 'La Peste dans la régence de Tunis aux XVIIe et XVIIIe siècles', *Revue de l'institut des belles lettres arabes*, 109 (1965), 48.

14 M. Kraiem, *La Tunisie précoloniale*, Vol. II (Tunis, 1973), pp. 355–7.

15 Lézine, *Deux villes*, p. 153.

16 L. Valensi, 'Calamités démographiques en Tunisie et en Méditerranée orientale aux XVIIIe et XIXe siècles', *Annales, E.S.C.*, 6 (November–December 1969), 1547.

17 Nyssen, cited in *ibid.*

18 Valensi, *Fellahs tunisiens*, p. 270.

19 Rousseau, cited in Plantet, *Correspondance*, III, p. 562. A consular letter written in December 1818 stated that at that time 250 to 500 were dying per day in Tunis and that the epidemic had begun in October 1817.

20 Devoise, cited in Valensi, 'Calamités démographiques', p. 1547.

21 Gallico, cited in *ibid.*, pp. 1156–7.

22 Valensi, *Fellahs tunisiens*, p. 284.

23 Bin Diyaf, VI, pp. 114–118.

24 *Safwat al-i'tibar*, p. 36.

25 Pellissier de Reynaud, quoted in Rouissi, 'Villes, villages', pp. 3–4.

26 Meyebire, quoted in *ibid.*, pp. 3–4.

27 Lumbroso, *Cenni sul cholera*, p. 231. Totals corrected by author.

28 *Ibid.*

29 J. Ganiage, *La Population européenne de Tunis au milieu du XIXe siècle* (Paris, 1960), p. 30.

30 Cotton, cited in F. Arnoulet, 'Histoire du choléra épidémique en Tunisie', *La Tunisie médicale*, 47, 6 (1969), 399–408. According to an ambassadorial report, all the European doctors but Cotton either left Tunis or refused to visit cholera patients during this epidemic. Ganiage, *La Population européenne*, p. 31, n. 38.

31 Ganiage, *La Population européenne*, p. 31.

32 H. Dunant, *La Régence de Tunis* (Tunis, 1875), p. 231.

33 Ganiage, *Origines*, p. 310; Ganiage, *La Population européenne*, p. 30.

34 Valensi, *Fellahs tunisiens*, p. 289. See also M. Rouissi, *Population et sociétés au Maghreb* (Tunis, 1978), pp. 35–76.

Glossary

'adl: juristic adjunct to a qāḍī, notary public
'ahd al-amān: in Tunisia, the constitution issued in 1857 and promulgated in 1860
ā'jamī: foreigner, non-Arab
'ālim: scholar, esp. in religious sciences (pl. 'ulamā')
'āmil: in Tunisia, administrative officer, head of an 'amāl (district)
amīn al-aṭibbā': chief doctor, head of doctors' order
amīr: ruler, prince, commander
amīr al-liwa': commanding officer, brigadier
amr: order or imperial decree, issued by an amīr
āya: verse from the Quran
baraka: magic property or special sense that brings about good fortune such as healing of disease
bāshā: pasha, Ottoman title for man of high rank
bāsh ḥakīm: chief or head doctor
bāsh kātib: chief or head secretary, scribe
bāsh ṭabīb: chief or head doctor
basmala: Muslim invocation ('in the name of God, the Merciful, the Compassionate')
bawwāb: doorman
bey: Ottoman military title; in Tunisia, title of ruler from 1705 to 1956
bū barak: father of kneeling
burnus: full-length hooded garment for men, usually woolen
bū shalal: father of paralysis
dey: Ottoman title; in Tunisia, title of ruler from 1591 to 1705
dhikr: invocation, repetition of words in praise of God
du'ā: invocation of God
fallaḥīn: peasants or farmers
funduq: hotel, caravanserai with rooms for merchandise and courtyard for animals
ghazwa: military expedition
ḥadīth: saying or deed of the Prophet or his companions, used as practical or legal guideline
ḥājib: protective device, amulet
ḥammām: public bath
Ḥanafi: one of four schools of Sharī'a law, followed by most Ottoman Turks

ḥāra: popular quarter of a city; in North Africa, Jewish quarter

ḥubus: waqf, habbous endowment

'īd: holiday, feast

ijāza: license or certificate of competence issued by a professional authority

imām: one who leads prayers in mosque services

Janissary: elite Ottoman soldier

jinn: invisible spirits, either harmful or helpful

kāhiya: deputy officer, replacement

kātib: scribe, secretary

khalīfa: successor; in Tunisia, provincial governor

khanduq: drain, ditch

khatm: protective seal, talisman

mabṭūn: afflicted with an intestinal ailment

madīna (or *medina*): city; now the *ancien ville* of Tunis, adjacent to the European sector

madrasa: school

maḥalla: in Tunisia, armed tax-collecting expedition

majba: tax; in nineteenth-century Tunisia, the 36-and 72- piaster head tax that set off the 1864 insurrection

majlis al-naẓāfa: Sanitary Service Committee (lit. Council of Cleanliness)

majlis al-taḥaffuẓ: Sanitary Council (lit. Council of Prevention [or Preservation])

makhzan: storehouse

Māliki: one of four schools of Sharī'a law, followed by most North and West Africans

ma'mal al-khubz: place where bread is made, bakery

mamlakata al-tūnisīyya: Kingdom of Tunis, name given to the Husayni state by Tunisian officials

Mamlūk: members of governing class, usually purchased in Caucasus or Greece, trained to fill high governmental or military positions

marabout (*murābit*, pl. *murabitūn*): in North Africa, saint or saint's tomb or shrine

maristān (ancient Persian: *bimaristan*): hospital, mental asylum

ma'ṣr al-zaytūn: place where olive oil is pressed

mawlid al-nabīy: birthday of the Prophet Muhammad

mu'adhdhin: one who gives the call to prayer, muezzin

mufti: official issuer of legal judgments under Islamic law

murabitūn: pl. of murābit (marabout)

mustashfā: hospital

naṣri: unit of money approximately equivalent to a riyal

nā'ūra: large, vertical water wheel

niẓām jadīd: nineteenth-century Muslim army trained by Europeans in European military style

qāḍī: religious judge

qafīz: unit of measurement approximately equal to 500 liters

qā'id (colloquial Tunisian: *gayd*): provincial authority, governor

Qaṣaba: citadel, site of government, Kasbah; now center of old city

rā'is al-dhabtīyya: chief of police

riyal: silver coin usually worth 20 piasters

ṣafsāri: shawl, often white silk or cotton, worn by women; sheet

ṣāḥib al-maḥalla: commander of the maḥalla

ṣāḥib al-ṭāba': keeper of the seal, minister of highest rank

sanjaq: Ottoman administrative province

ṣaqīfa: vestibule, entryway opening to courtyard

shahada: Muslim profession of faith ('there is no god but God and Muhammad is his Prophet')

shahid: witness

Sharī'a: the revealed law of Islam

sharīf: descendant of the Prophet Muhammad

shāshīya: felt cap worn in North Africa, often called fez or tarboush

shaykh: senior authority, religious dignitary, master

shaykh al-madīna: city guardian or mayor of Tunis appointed by the bey

Si, Sidi: in North Africa, Mister or Sir; also Said or Sayyid in classical Arabic

Ṣūfi: Islamic mystic, member of religious order

sūq: market, bazaar

sūra: chapter of the Quran

ṭabaqāt: biographical notes

ṭabīb: doctor

takīya: hospice of religious (Ṣūfi) order

tanzimāt: series of Ottoman governmental reforms undertaken in the nineteenth century

tasbīḥ: blessing or glorification of God

tirfas: truffle, underground fungus that produces edible tubers

'ulamā': pl. of 'ālim

al-wabā' al-kabīr: the Great Epidemic (wabā' at the time customarily meant plague)

wakīl: manager, trustee

waqf: religious endowment, inalienable property prescribed by Islamic law

wazīr al-akbār: prime minister

wazīr al-'amāla: minister of the interior

wazīr al-māl: minister of finance

zāwiya: in North Africa, small mosque built over the tomb of a saint, often with teaching facilities and a hospice; usually associated with Ṣūfi order

Bibliography

I. Public archival collections

Archives Générales du Gouvernement Tunisien [A.G.G.T.], Dar al-Bey, Ministry of Foreign Affairs, Tunis.

Public Record Office, correspondence between British consuls in Tunis and Foreign Office [F.O.], London.

Middle East Centre, St Antony's College, Oxford, Richard Wood papers.

II. Newspapers

Gazette médicale de Paris. Paris.
Journal officiel tunisien. Tunis.
La Presse. Tunis.
Nuzhat al-khayriyya, the government almanac. Tunis, 1870–80.
Ra'id al-tunisi. Tunis.

III. General works on medicine and public health

Ackerknecht, E. 'Anticontagionism between 1821 and 1867'. *Bulletin of the History of Medicine*, 22 (1948), 562–93.

A Short History of Medicine, New York, 1968.

Bennassar, B. *Recherches sur les grandes épidémies dans le nord de l'Espagne à la fin du XVIe siècle: problèmes de documentation et de méthode*. Paris, 1969.

Biraben, J.N. 'Les Conceptions médico-épidémiologiques actuelles de la peste'. *Le Concours médical* (26 January 1957), 619–25.

Les Hommes et la peste en France et dans les pays européens et méditerranéens. 2 vols. Paris, 1975–6.

'La Peste dans l'Europe occidentale et le bassin méditerranéen: principales épidémies, conceptions médicales, moyens de lutte'. *Le Concours médical* (2 February 1963), 781–90.

Bowsky, W., ed. *The Black Death: A Turning Point in History?* New York, 1971.

Brieger, G. *Medical America in the Nineteenth Century*. Baltimore, 1972.

Briggs, A. 'Cholera and Society in the Nineteenth Century'. *Past and Present*, 19 (1961), 76–96.

Brockway, L. *Science and Colonial Expansion: The Role of the British Royal Botanical Gardens*. New York, 1979.

Burnet, M., and D. White. *Natural History of Infectious Disease*. Cambridge, 1972.

Cahill, ed. *The Untapped Resource: Medicine and Diplomacy*. New York, 1971.

Carpentier, E. 'Autour de la peste noire: famines et épidémies dans l'histoire du XIVe siècle'. *Annales E.S.C.*, 17, 2 (1962), 1062–92.

Une ville devant la peste: Orvieto et la peste noire de 1348. Paris, 1962.

Chevalier, L. *Le Choléra: la première épidémie du XIXe siècle*. La Roche-sur-Yon, 1958.

Classes laborieuses et classes dangereuses à Paris pendant la première moitié du XIXe siècle. Paris, 1958.

Cipolla, C. *Cristofano and the Plague: A Study in the History of Public Health in the Age of Galileo*. Berkeley, 1973.

The Economic History of World Populations. Baltimore, 1962.

Faith, Reason, and the Plague in Seventeenth-Century Tuscany. Ithaca, 1979.

Public Health and the Medical Profession in the Renaissance. New York, 1976.

Clarke, E., ed. *Modern Methods in the History of Medicine*. London, 1971.

Defoe, D. *A Journal of the Plague Year*. London, 1722.

Dubos, R. *Man Adapting*. New Haven, 1965.

Foucault, M. *Birth of the Clinic*. New York, 1973.

Haggard, H. *Devils, Drugs, and Doctors*. New York and London, 1929.

Hirst, L. *The Conquest of Plague: A Study of the Evolution of Epidemiology*. Oxford, 1953.

Hobson, W. *The Theory and Practice of Public Health*. London, 1975.

Howard-Jones, N. 'Cholera Therapy in the Nineteenth Century'. *Journal of the History of Medicine*, 27, 4 (October 1972), 373–95.

Illich, I. *Medical Nemesis: The Expropriation of Health*. New York, 1976.

King, L. *The Medical World of the Eighteenth Century*. Chicago, 1958.

Langer, W. 'The Next Assignment'. *The American Historical Review*, 23, 2 (January 1958), 283–304.

McGrew, R. *Russia and the Cholera*. Madison, 1965.

McNeill, W. *Plagues and Peoples: A History*. New York, 1976.

May, J. *The Ecology of Human Disease*. New York, 1958.

Pelling, M. *Cholera, Fever, and English Medicine, 1825–1865*. Oxford, 1978.

Pollitzer, R. *Cholera*. Geneva, 1959.

Post, J. 'Famine, Mortality, and Epidemic Disease in the Process of Modernization'. *Economic History Review*, 21, 1 (1976), 14–37.

Prus, R. *Rapport à l'académie royale de médecine sur la peste et les quarantines*. 2 vols. Paris, 1846.

le Riche, W., and J. Milner. *Epidemiology as Medical Ecology*. Edinburgh, 1884.

Rosen, G. *A History of Public Health*. New York, 1958.

'People, Disease, and Emotion: Some Newer Problems for Research in Medical History'. *Bulletin of the History of Medicine*, 41 (January–February 1967), 5–23.

Rosenberg, C. *The Cholera Years: The United States in 1832, 1849, and 1866*. Chicago, 1962.

Shrewsbury, J. *A History of Bubonic Plague in the British Isles*. Cambridge, 1970.

Sigerist, H. *Civilization and Disease.* Chicago, 1962.
   Medicine and Human Welfare. New Haven, 1941.
Snow, J. *Snow on Cholera.* New York, 1936.
Susser, M. *Causal Thinking in the Health Sciences: Concepts and Strategies of Epidemiology.* New York, 1973.
Trevelyan, G. *English Social History: A Survey of Six Centuries, Chaucer to Queen Victoria.* London, 1943.
Winslow, C. *The Conquest of Epidemic Disease: A Chapter in the History of Ideas.* Princeton, 1943.
   Man and Epidemics. Princeton, 1952.
Ziegler, P. *The Black Death.* New York, 1969.
Zinsser, H. *Rats, Lice, and History.* New York, 1971.

IV. Works on North Africa and the Middle East

Abdesselem, Ahmad. *Les Historiens tunisiens des XVIIe, XVIIIe, et XIXe siècles.* Paris, 1971.
Abun-Nasr, J. *A History of the Maghrib.* Cambridge, 1971.
   The Tijaniyya: A Sufi Order in the Modern World. London, 1965.
Adivar, Adnan. *La Science chez les Turcs ottomans.* Paris, 1939.
Ammad, Sleim. *En souvenir de la médecine arabe: quelques-uns de ses grands noms.* Tunis, 1965.
al-Antaki, Da'ud. *Tadhkirat uli al-albab wa al-jami' al-ajab al-ujab.* Cairo, 1885–6.
Arnoulet, F. 'Le Choléra épidémique en Tunisie'. Doct. d'état, médecine. Paris, 1948.
   'Histoire du choléra épidémique en Tunisie'. *La Tunisie médicale,* 47, 6 (1969), 399–411.
al-Bayluni, Fath Allah. 'Khulasat ma tahsul 'alayhi al-sa'un fi adwiyat dafa' al-waba' wa al-ta'un'. MS. U.C.L.A. Ar. 6 i.
Bayram al-Khamis, M. *al-Hammamat al-ma'daniya.* Cairo, 1906.
   Safwat al-i'tibar bi mustawda al-amsar wa al-aqtar. Vol. II, Bk 2. Beirut, 1972–3.
Bdira, M. *Relations internationales et sous-développement: la Tunisie, 1857–1864.* Uppsala, 1978.
Ben Milad, Ahmad. *L'École médicale de Kairouan aux Xe et XIe siècles.* Paris, 1933. *See also* Ibn Milad, Ahmad.
Berbrugger, L. *Mémoire sur la peste en Algérie, 1552–1819.* Paris, 1847.
Berque, J. *L'Intérieur du Maghreb, XVe–XIXe siècles.* Paris, 1978.
Bertherand, E. *Médecine et hygiène des Arabes.* Paris, 1855.
Bin Diyaf, Ahmad. *See* Ibn Abi Diyaf, Ahmad.
al-Bistami, 'Abd al-Rahman. 'Wasf al-dawa' fi kashf afat al-waba''. MS. U.C.L.A. Ar. 21 iv.
Bloch, E. 'Peste d'alors et d'aujourd'hui'. *La Tunisie médicale,* 24 (1930), 17–27.
   La Peste en Tunisie: aperçu historique et épidémiologique. Tunis, 1929.
Bois, C. 'Années de disette, années d'abondance, sécheresse et pluies en Tunisie de 648 à 1881'. *Revue sur l'étude des calamités* (Geneva, 1944), 3–26.
Bousquet, G. *L'Islam maghrebin.* Algiers, 1954.

Braudel, F. *La Méditerranée et le monde méditerranéen à l'époque de Philippe II.* 2 vols. Paris, 1966.

Brown, K. 'On the Appropriation of Surplus in Tunisia since the Nineteenth Century'. *Dialectical Anthropology*, 4, 1 (1979), 57–64.

Brown, L.C. *The Tunisia of Ahmad Bey, 1837–1855.* Princeton, 1974.

Browne, E. *Arabian Medicine.* Cambridge, 1921.

Brunel, R. *Essai sur la confrérie religieuse des 'Aissaoua au Maroc.* Paris, 1926.

Brunschvig, R. *La Berberie orientale sous les Hafsides.* 2 vols. Paris, 1940 and 1946.

'Justice religieuse et justice laïque dans la Tunisie des deys et des beys, jusqu'au milieu du XIXe siècle'. *Studia Islamica*, 23 (1965), 27–70.

Bukhari, M. *Sahih al-Bukhari.* Cairo, 1966.

Cambon, H. *Histoire de la régence de Tunis.* Paris, 1948.

Cherif, Ahmad. 'Histoire de la médecine arabe en Tunisie'. Doct. d'état, médecine. Bordeaux, 1908.

Cherif, M.H. *L'Ankylose de l'économie méditerranéenne au XVIIIe et au début du XIXe siècle : le rôle de l'agriculture.* Nice, 1973.

'Les Domaines de l'histoire : l'expansion européenne et difficultés tunisiennes de 1815 à 1830'. *Annales, E.S.C.*, 3, 25 (1970), 714–45.

Conor, M. 'Une épidémie de peste en Afrique mineure (1784–1788)'. *Archives de l'institut Pasteur de Tunis*, 2 (1911), 220–41.

Conseil, E. 'Médecine tunisienne d'hier : rapport sur l'épidémie du choléra en 1911'. *La Tunisie médicale*, 6 (July–August 1970), 221–41.

Crapanzano, V. *The Hamadsha : A Study in Moroccan Ethnopsychiatry.* London, 1973.

Cubisol, C. *Notices abrégées sur la régence de Tunis.* Bone, 1867.

De Kay, J. *Sketches of Turkey in 1831 and 1832.* New York, 1833.

Demeerseman, A. 'Licences d'exportation d'huile tunisienne, 1816–1823'. *Revue de l'institut des belles lettres arabes*, 137, 1 (1976), 73–119.

Dessort, C. *L'Histoire de la ville de Tunis.* Algiers, 1924.

Dinguizli, B. 'Aperçu rétrospectif sur l'exercice de la profession médicale et de l'assistance médicale en Tunisie avant l'occupation française dans ce pays'. *La Tunisie médicale*, special edn (May 1931), 177–83.

Dols, M. *The Black Death in the Middle East.* Princeton, 1977.

Doutté, E. *Magie et religion dans l'Afrique du nord.* Algiers, 1909.

Dunant, H. *La Régence de Tunis.* Tunis, 1975.

Elgood, C. *A Medical History of Persia and the Eastern Caliphate.* Cambridge, 1951.

Safavid Medical Practice. London, 1971.

d'Estournelles de Constant [P.H.X.]. *La Politique française en Tunisie : le protectorat et ses origines, 1854–1891.* Paris, 1891.

Ferrini, G. *Intorno al cholera di Tunisi dell'anno 1867.* Milan, 1868.

Saggio sul clima e sulle principal malattie della citta di Tunisi e del regno. Milan, 1860.

Fisher, H. 'Hassebu : Islamic Healing in Black Africa'. In M. Brett, ed., *Northern Africa : Islam and Modernization*, pp. 23–48. London, 1973.

de Flaux, A. *La Régence de Tunis au dix-neuvième siècle.* Paris, 1865.

Frank, L. 'Tunis'. In *L'Univers, histoire et description de tous les peuples : Algérie, Etats Tripolitains, Tunis*, pp. 3–143. Paris, 1850.

Gallagher, N. 'The Arab Medical Organization in Nineteenth-Century Tunisia'. *Revue d'histoire maghrebine*, 4 (July 1975), 145–9.

Gandolphe, M. 'Notes inédites sur Tunisie en 1786 et sur son épidémie de peste en 1785, extraites du journal de Père Vicheret'. *Revue tunisienne*, 25 (1918), 214–21.

'Premiers hôpitaux français en Tunisie'. *La Tunisie médicale*, special edn (May 1931), 167–70.

Ganiage, J. *Les Origines du protectorat français en Tunisie, 1863–1881*. Paris, 1959.

'La Population de la Tunisie vers 1860: essai d'évaluation d'après les registres fiscaux'. *Population*, 21, 5 (September–October 1966), 857–86.

La Population européenne de Tunis au milieu du XIXe siècle. Paris, 1960.

Gilsenan, M. *Saint and Sufi in Modern Egypt : An Essay in the Sociology of Religions*. New York, 1973.

Gomma, F. *L'Assistance médicale en Tunisie : essai sur l'histoire de la médecine et de l'hygiène publique dans la régence*. Tunis, 1904.

Grandchamp, P. *Documents relatifs à la révolution de 1864 en Tunisie*. 2 vols. Tunis, 1935.

Documents relatifs aux corsaires tunisiens, 1777–1824. Tunis, 1925.

Etudes d'histoire tunisienne, XVIIe–XXe siècles. Paris, 1966.

Greenwood, B. 'Ambiguity of Illness Classification in a Pluralistic Medical System: A Moroccan Example'. MS. London, 1980.

Guyon, J. 'Lettre sur l'état du choléra dans la régence de Tunis'. *Gazette médicale de Paris*, 3rd ser., 5 (1850), 401.

L'Histoire des épidémies du nord de l'Afrique depuis les temps les plus reculés jusqu'à nos jours. Algiers, 1955.

Hamarneh, S. *Fihris makhtutat dar al-kutub al-zahiriyya : al-tibb wa al-saydala*. Damascus, 1969.

Hartwig, G., ed. *Disease in African History*. Durham, N.C., 1978.

Hilton-Simpson, M. *Arab Medicine and Surgery : A Study of the Healing Art in Algeria*. London, 1922.

Hugon, H. *Les Emblèmes des beys de Tunis*. Paris, 1913.

Ibn 'Abd al-'Aziz, Hamuda. *Kitab al-bashi*. Pt I, Tunis, 1970; complete MSS Nos. 1236 and 1249, British Museum.

Ibn Abi Dinar, M. *al-Mu'nis fi akhbar ifriqiya wa tunis*. Tunis, 1976.

Ibn Abi Diyaf [Bin Diyaf], Ahmad. 'Chronicle of the Reign of Ahmad Bey'. In Ahmed Abdesselem, ed., *Ithaf ahl al-zaman bi akhbar muluk tunis wa 'ahd al-aman*, Ch. 6. Tunis, 1971.

Ithaf ahl al-zaman bi akhbar muluk tunis wa 'ahd al-aman. 8 vols. Tunis, 1963–6.

Ibn Ashur, M. *al-Haraka al-adabiya wa al-fikriya fi tunis*. Cairo, 1956.

Ibn Kamal, Ahmad. 'Risalah al-waba'iya'. MS. U.C.L.A. Ar. 22 iv and v.

Ibn Milad, Ahmad. 'Mustashfayat bi-tunis'. 3 pts. *Fikr*, 18, 3 (December 1972), 63–7; 19, 1 (October 1973), 50–4; 19, 5 (February 1974), 62–7. *See also* Ben Milad, Ahmad.

Ibn al-Mubarak, Husayn. *al-Tajdid al-sahih*. Beirut, n.d.

Issawi, C. 'British Trade and the Rise of Beirut, 1830–1860'. *International Journal of Middle East Studies*, 8, 1 (January 1977), 91–101.

Johnson, P. 'A Sufi Shrine in Tunisia'. Ph.D. dissertation. Berkeley, 1979.

Julien, C.-A. *History of North Africa*. London, 1970.

Kennedy, J. *Algeria and Tunis in 1845*. 2 vols. London, 1846.

al-Khuja, M. 'Wathiqa tarikhiya jalila'. *al-Majallat al-zaytuna* (October 1939), 374–91.

Klein, C.H. 'Changing Health Beliefs and Practices in an Urban Setting: A Tunisian Example'. Ph.D. dissertation. New York, 1975.

Kraiem, M. *La Tunisie précoloniale*. 2 vols. Tunis, 1973.

Kuhnke, L. 'Resistance and Response to Modernization: Preventive Medicine and Social Control in Egypt, 1825–1850'. Ph.D. dissertation. Chicago, 1971.

Ladjimi, M. 'L'Empirisme médical chez les musulmans tunisiens'. Doct. d'état médecine. Lyon, 1920.

Laroui, A. *L'Histoire du Maghreb: un essai de synthèse*. Paris, 1970.

Legy, F. *The Folklore of Morocco*. London, 1935.

Leslie, C., ed. *Asian Medical Systems: A Comparative Study*. Berkeley, 1976.

Levi-Provençal, E. *Les Historiens des Chorfa*. Paris, 1922.

Lewis, B. *The Muslim Discovery of Europe*. New York, 1982.

Lézine, A. *Deux villes d'Ifriqiyya*. Paris, 1971.

Liauzu, C. 'Les Libertaires en Tunisie'. *Cahiers de Tunisie*, 21 (1973), 157–82.

Limam, R. 'Siyasa hamuda basha al-husayni fi al-mahal al-tijari'. *Revue d'histoire maghrebine*, 2 (July 1974), 83–8.

Loir, A. 'Démographie–statistique de la population de Tunis'. *Revue tunisienne*, 19 (1898), 348–54.

'L'Hygiène'. In *La Tunisie: histoire et description*, Vol. 1, pp. 193–205. Paris, 1896.

Loth, G. *Le Peuplement italien en Tunisie et en Algérie*. Tunis, 1905.

Lovy, F. 'L'Hôpital Sadiki de 1893 à 1902'. *La Tunisie médicale*, special edn (May 1931), 207–70.

'Notes sur la vie médicale à Tunis avant l'occupation'. *La Tunisie médicale*, special edn (May 1931), 209–17.

Lumbroso, A. *Cenni storico-scientifici sul cholera-morbus asiatico che invase la reggenza di Tunis nel 1849–1850*. Marseilles, 1850.

Lettres médico-statistiques sur la régence de Tunis. Marseilles, 1860.

Magnin, J. 'Médecine d'hier et médecins d'aujourd'hui'. *Revue de l'institut des belles lettres arabes*, 80 (1957), 393–416.

Malinas, M., and M. Tostivint. 'Mutualité coopérative et projet général d'assistance médicale indigène'. *Revue tunisienne*, 12 (1905), 283–304, 386–422, 480–515.

Ma'oz, M. *Ottoman Reform in Syria and Palestine, 1840–1861*. Oxford, 1968.

Marchika, J. *La Peste en Afrique septentrionale*. Algiers, 1927.

Masson, P. *Histoire des établissements et du commerce français dans l'Afrique barbaresque, 1560–1793*. Paris, 1903.

Matignon, J. *L'Art médical à Tunis*. Paris, 1901.

Molco, E. 'L'Art médical en Tunisie avant le protectorat'. *La Tunisie médicale*, special edn (May 1931), 184–206.

Monchicourt, C. *Documents historiques sur la Tunisie : relations inédites de Nyssen, Filippi et Calligaris, 1788, 1829, 1834*. Paris, 1929.

Montague, J. 'Notes on Medical Organization in Nineteenth Century Tunisia: A Preliminary Analysis of the Materials on Public Health and Medicine in the Dar el Bey in Tunis'. *Medical History*, 17, 1 (January 1973), 75–82.

Mzali, M. *L'Hérédité dans la dynastie husseinite*. Tunis, 1969.

Nachtigal, G. *Sahara und Soudan*. Berlin, 1879. A. Fisher and H. Fisher, trans. Berkeley, 1971.

Nasr, Hossein. *Islamic Science*. Westerham, Kent, 1976.

al-Nasr, M. *Tarikh jirba*. Tunis, n.d.

Neveu, R. 'L'Etat sanitaire de l'Afrique du nord pendant l'occupation arabo-turque'. *Société française d'histoire de la médecine française*, 12 (1912), 407–521.

Nunes-Vais, G. *Studi clinici sul cholera*. Tunis, 1885.

Paul, J. 'Medicine and Imperialism in Morocco'. *Middle East Research and Information Project Reports*, 60 (September 1977), 3–12.

Pellegrin, A. *Le Vieux Tunis : les noms des rues de la ville arabe*. Tunis, 1955.

Pellissier de Reynaud, E. *Description de la régence de Tunis, exploration scientifique de l'Algérie*. Vol. 6. Paris, 1853.

Perussel, Docteur. 'L'Assistance des psychopathes en Tunisie'. *La Tunisie médicale*, special edn (May 1931), 277–84.

Peyssonnel, J.A., and R.L. Desfontaines. *Voyages dans les régences de Tunis et d'Alger*. 2 vols. Paris, 1838.

Plantet, E. *Correspondance des beys de Tunis et des consuls de France avec la cour, 1577–1830*. 3 vols. Paris, 1893–9.

Poiret, Abbé. *Voyage en Barbarie, ou lettres écrites de l'ancienne Numidia pendant les années de 1785 et 1786*. 2 vols. Paris, 1789.

Raymond, A. 'Les Grandes Epidémies de peste au Caire aux XVIIe et XVIIIe siècles'. *Bulletin d'études orientales*, 25 (1972), 203–10.

'Les Porteurs d'eau de Caire'. *Institut français d'archéologie orientale*, 56–7 (1957–8), 183–202.

'Signes urbains et études de la population des grandes villes arabes à l'époque ottomane'. *Bulletin d'études orientales*, 27 (1974), 183–93.

Reynaud, L. 'Recherches historiques sur les épidémies du Maroc, au XVIIIe siècle'. *Hesperis*, 24 (1939), 293–319.

'Recherches historiques sur les épidémies du Maroc: la peste de 1799 d'après les documents inédits'. *Hesperis*, 1 (1921), 160–82.

'Recherches historiques sur les épidémies du Maroc: la peste de 1818 au Maroc'. *Hesperis*, 3 (1923), 13–36.

Rinn, L. *Marabouts et Khouan : étude sur l'islam en Algérie*. Algiers, 1884.

Robson, J. *Mishkat al-masabih*. Vol. III. Lahore, 1964.

Rouissi, M. *Population et sociétés au Maghreb*. Tunis, 1978.

'Villes, villages, et tribes de Tunisie à la fin du XIXe siècle'. Unpublished paper.

Rousseau, A. *Annales tunisiennes, ou aperçu historique sur la régence de Tunis.* Algiers, 1864.

de Saint-Gervais. *Mémoires historiques que concernent le gouvernement de l'ancien et du nouveau royaume de Tunis.* Paris, 1736.

al-Sanusi al-Hasani, Yusuf. *Mujarrabat al-dirbiy al-kabir.* Tunis, n.d.

Sebag, P. 'Une description de Tunis au XIXe siècle'. *Cahiers de Tunisie,* 6–7 (1959), 161–81.

'La Peste dans la régence de Tunis aux XVIIe et XVIIIe siècles'. *Revue de l'institut des belles lettres arabes,* 109 (1965), 35–48.

Seghir ben Youssef, M. *Mechra et Melki: chronique tunisienne,* 1705–1771. Tunis, 1900.

Şehsuvaroğlu, B. *Tarihi kolera salginlare ve oslanle turkleri.* Istanbul, 1954.

Seklani, M. *La Population de la Tunisie.* Tunis, 1974.

Sfar, B. *Assistance publique musulmane en Tunis.* Tunis, 1896.

Shah, M. *The General Principles of Avicenna's Canon.* Karachi, 1966.

Shaw, T. *Travels and Observations Relating to Several Parts of Barbary and Levant.* Oxford, 1738.

Slama, B. *L'Insurrection de 1864 en Tunisie.* Tunis, 1967.

Sublet, J. 'La Peste prise aux rets de la jurisprudence: le traité d'Ibn Hagar al 'Asqalani sur la peste'. *Studia Islamica,* 33 (1971), 141–9.

al-Suyuti, Jalal al-Din. 'Ma rawahu al-waun fi akhbar al-ta'un'. MS. U.C.L.A. Ar. 2 i.

al-Rahma fi al-tibb wa al-hikma. Tunis, n.d.

'Tibb-ul-nabbi or Medicine of the Prophet'. C. Elgood, trans. *Osiris,* 14 (1962), 33–192.

Thabit Ibn Qurra, al-Sabi. *The Book of al Dakhira (Kitab al-dakhira fi 'ilm al-tibb).* G. Sobhy, ed. Cairo, 1928.

Tlili, B. *Etudes d'histoire sociale tunisienne du XIXe siècle.* Tunis, 1974.

le Tourneau, R. *Les Villes musulmanes de l'Afrique du nord.* Algiers, 1957.

al-Tunisi, Khayr al-Din. *The Surest Path.* L.C. Brown, trans. Cambridge, 1967.

Turin, Y. *Affrontements culturels dans l'Algérie coloniale: écoles, médecines, religion, 1830–1880.* Paris, 1971.

Vaidon, L. *Tangier: A Different Way.* Metuchen, N.J., 1977.

Valensi, L. 'Calamités démographiques en Tunisie et en Méditerranée orientale aux XVIIIe et XIXe siècles'. *Annales, E.S.C.,* 6 (November–December 1969), 1540–62.

'La Conjoncture agaire en Tunisie aux XVIIIe et XIXe siècles'. *Revue historique,* 494 (April–June 1970), 321–36.

Fellahs tunisiens: l'économie rurale et la vie des campagnes aux XVIIIe et XIXe siècles. Paris, 1977.

'Islam et capitalisme: production et commerce des chechias en Tunisie et en France aux XVIIIe et XIXe siècles'. *Revue d'histoire moderne et contemporaine,* 16 (1969), 376–400.

Le Maghreb avant la prise d'Alger. Paris, 1969.

'Le Maghreb précolonial: mode de production archaïque ou mode de production féodale?' In collaboration with R. Galissot, *La Pensée* (December 1968), 57–93.

'Les Relations commerciales entre la régence de Tunis et Malte au XVIIIe siècle'. *Cahiers de Tunisie*, 43 (1963), 71–83.

'The Tunisian Fellaheen in the Eighteenth and Nineteenth Centuries'. In A. Udovitch, ed., *The Islamic Middle East, 700–1900: Studies in Economic and Social History*, pp. 704–24. Princeton, 1981.

Valensi, L., and M. Ben Smail. 'Le Régne de Hammuda Pacha dans la chronique d'Ibn Abi Diyaf'. *Cahiers de Tunisie*, 73–4 (1973–4), 87–108.

Wensinck, A. *Concordance et indices de la tradition musulmane.* 7 vols. Leiden, 1936–69.

Westermarck, E. *Ritual and Belief in Morocco.* 2 vols. London, 1926.

Yacono, X. 'Peut-on évaluer la population de l'Algérie vers 1830?' *Revue africaine*, 98 (1954), 277–307.

Index

'Abd Allah b. Muhammad b. Muhammad
  b. Muhammad Bayram III, 31
Abu 'Abd Allah Muhammad Basha, see
  Hamuda Basha al-Muradi
Abu 'Abd Allah Muhammad Sulayman b.
  al-Mana'i, 31
'ahd al-aman (Fundamental Pact) , 65
Ahmad Bey, 43–8, 51–5, 61–3, 83, 98
agriculture, recession in, 36–7, 38, 123
  n. 5
'Ali Bey, 15–16, 19, 22, 24, 25, 34, 94
allopathy, 88
amin al-atibba's, 17, 21, 82, 83, 87, 101
al-Antaki, Da'ud, 27, 29
al-'Arbi Zarruq, 64, 90
astral influences, as suspected cause of
  epidemic disease, 11, 29
'Aziza 'Uthmana, 22, 91

Bayram al-Khamis, 67, 75, 80–1, 90,
  109–10
Behçet, Mustafa, 58–9
Bertherand, Dr E., 22, 56
Bin Ahmad, Qaddur, 87, 94
Bin Diyaf (Ibn Abi Diyaf), Ahmad
  accounts of epidemics: cholera
    (1849–50), 49, 52–3, 62, 63, (1867)
    69–77; famine (1866), 66, 67–8;
    plague (1818–20), 31–3, 38; typhus
    (1868), 78–81
  and 'ahd al-aman (Fundamental Pact),
    65
  attitude to quarantine, 52–3, 60
  on population decline, 109–10
Black Death (1348), 7

Castelnuovo, Dr Giacomo, 46, 89, 90, 92,
  99
cautery, 9
Chirac, Dr M., 11
cholera
  descriptive background, 5–6

epidemics (1836), 42–3, (1849–50)
  46–59, (1856) 59–60, 130 n. 30,
  (1867) 69–77, 126 n. 62
mortality (1849–50), 53–4, 55, 59,
  110–12, (1867) 73, 81, 82
remedies: European, 57–9, 76; Muslim,
  56–7, 76
Clot Bey, 12, 53–4
contagion, see quarantine
Cotton, Dr, 44, 57, 69, 112, 130 n. 30
Curillo, Dr Joseph (Yusuf al-Qurir), 19,
  116 n. 14

Desfontaines, Dr R. L., 16, 19, 29–30
Dinguizli, Bechir, 87, 94
doctors
  European, 19–20, 47–8, 51–2, 54, 57,
    70–2, 76, 82, 83–8, 93–6, 100–1; chief
    physicians at court, 128 n. 17;
    empirical practitioners, 88–90;
    political–commercial role, 19, 88, 99,
    127–8 n. 15
  Muslim, 16–19, 21, 56, 76, 83–8, 93–6,
    100–1
  Ottoman: Muslim 58–9, 116 n. 18;
    non-Muslim, 20–1, 116 n. 18

epidemics, see cholera, plague, typhus
Europeans, in Tunis, 28–9, 30, 68, 75–6,
  78–9, 88, 123 n. 13; see also doctors

fatalism, 25–6, 30, 31–2, 52–4, 73, 96,
  100–1, 119 n. 3
Ferrini, Dr G., 57, 76
Filippi, Count, 22, 115 n. 7
Frank, Dr Louis, 1, 17, 19, 117 n. 51

Galenic–Islamic medicine, 7–8, 9, 11, 13,
  20, 88
germ theory, 12–13

Hamda b. Kilani, 1, 17, 87, 93

143

For EU product safety concerns, contact us at Calle de José Abascal, 56–1°,
28003 Madrid, Spain or eugpsr@cambridge.org.

www.ingramcontent.com/pod-product-compliance
Ingram Content Group UK Ltd.
Pitfield, Milton Keynes, MK11 3LW, UK
UKHW010854090126
466816UK00011B/242